When Living Alone Means Living at Risk

Golden Age Books

Perspectives on Aging

Series Editor: Steven L. Mitchell

When Living Alone Means Living at Risk

A Guide for Caregivers and Families

edited by

Robert W. Buckingham, Dr. P.H.

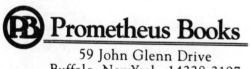 Prometheus Books

59 John Glenn Drive
Buffalo, NewYork 14228-2197

Published 1994 by Prometheus Books

98 97 96 95 94   5 4 3 2 1

Library of Congress Cataloging-in-Publication Data

Buckingham, Robert W.
    When living alone means living at risk : a guide for caregivers and families
edited by Robert W. Buckingham.
        p.   cm. — (Golden age books)
    Includes bibliographical references.
    ISBN 0-87975-844-9 (cloth) — ISBN 0-87975-873-2 (pbk.)
    1. Aged—Health and hygiene. 2. Aged—Medical Care. 3. Aged—Care.
4. Caregivers—Mental Health. 5. Aged—Family relationships. I. Title.
II. Series.
RA564.8.B83   1994
362.1'9897—dc20   93-33990
                                                               CIP

Printed in the United States of America on acid-free paper.

To

Bill Faraclas,

my dear friend and brother

Contents

8   Contents

Introduction

Robert W. Buckingham, Dr. P. H.

In recent years there have been many books, articles, television news programs, and open public forums devoted to the needs of our nation's elders: how to improve the public's perception of the elderly and increase our awareness of the aging process, the state of healthcare in general and long-term care in particular, housing, assistive services, and other important topics. As a nation, we want to help our older citizens live long and enjoyable lives in the hope that they will continue to contribute to society's rich and diverse texture.

To achieve these broad social goals, experts in many fields have suggested public policies, social service strategies, and care-related programs to make it possible for the elderly to remain in their communities for as long as seems practical based upon their individual wishes and the relative state of their health. But while this is an admirable objective, America has changed in ways that make these goals much harder to realize.

Ours is a highly mobile society with children often living many miles away from their parents. The close familial unit that was so much a part of traditional American life and, in part, a function of sheer physical proximity has been dealt a serious blow (if not totally shattered) by decades of high divorce rates; more and more adult children choosing to postpone major life commitments in order to remain flexible with respect to employment prospects; and the stresses and strains of an economy that is working its way through a post-Cold War era in which global competition, scarce resources, and the demands of healthcare and other urgent social needs find local, state, and federal governments strained to the limit. The established patterns of social and familial behavior have changed, and our nation finds itself facing the twenty-first century wondering how the young and the old alike will confront a host of divisive issues.

The effort to encourage elders to maintain active and meaningful lives in the community is admirable and, in the long run, far more cost effective than placing increasing numbers of individuals in expensive residential facilities or in skilled-care nursing homes. But in many ordinary, pleasant, and otherwise comfortable streets throughout America there can be found elders who live alone and are at risk of serious physical and/or emotional harm. What of the older gentleman who lives two doors down, but none of his neighbors have seen him for days? They worry about him because he doesn't answer his phone or come to the door. And what of the frail old woman in the big house who seems barely able to move about the place yet she fears that if she accepts help, her family will think she can no longer take care of herself and will rush her off to an "old folks home"? Then there are the elders who have trouble seeing or hearing clearly or who are unsteady of gait and run the risk of serious falls. How are we to address the aging man or woman who experiences moderate to deep depressions or other psychological problems, which render them disinterested in eating properly, taking their medications, or maintaining good hygiene?

To be of help to America's aging population, family members, friends, social service providers, and other concerned persons must not only be willing to separate their private views on aging and their personal attitudes about what constitutes an enjoyable, fulfilling life from the views and attitudes held by their elderly loved ones; they must also be mindful of the need to respect the autonomy and choices of aged relatives and friends, even if they disagree with the decisions these elders might make. How are concerned people to help the elders in their lives while at the same time recognizing that even though many old people are or appear to be in desperate need of a helping hand, their right to live as they choose within the limits of their capacities must be respected, encouraged, admired, and supported? Caregivers, social service providers, families, and friends need to appreciate the uniqueness of each individual elder while making every effort to ease the frustration that older people feel when routine physical tasks are too hard to perform, the anxiety that overcomes them when they can't remember whether they have taken needed medications on time, and the confusion and fear that accompanies diminished sight and/or hearing. The physical, emotional, financial, and psychological obstacles facing today's elders are significant, and the defenses they have set up to protect themselves from the pain of life often leave casual observers with the impression that many older people are cranky, difficult, opinionated, eccentric, unpredictable, out of sorts, or disagreeable. But before we succumb to a stereotyped and jaded view of the elderly, we must ask ourselves how well we could adjust to the many traumatic situations in which thousands of older Americans find themselves every day.

I have organized this book around the medical, social, and psychological concerns that affect our elders. No one volume could address all the relevant issues, but here readers will be met with some of the major practical problems confronted daily by a great many older people who live alone. Certainly such issues as the uncooperative elder (chapter 1); drug misuse, whether over- or undermedication (chapter 2); financial concerns (chapter 3); and the importance of nutrition (chapter 4) have been the fodder for newspaper columns, magazine stories, and prime-time television news programs. The contributors to this volume have made every effort to address each issue head-on. For example, chapters 5, 6, and 7 focus on the physical challenges of vision loss, hearing loss, and reduced mobility. The limitations such diminished capacity poses would frighten anyone but these physical obstacles afflict the elderly in far greater numbers. In each area we have tried to provide skills and adaptive behavior to successfully cope with these challenges.

The importance of excercise for elders (chapter 8) has only recently been brought to the public's attention. As elders experience the benefits of walking, jogging, and low-impact aerobics, the combination of proper nutrition (a diet low in fat and high in complex carbohydrates) and a daily exercise routine should begin to decrease the physical and emotional risks they face, while increasing their sense of well-being.

Regrettably, the pages of newspapers and magazines are filled with stories of the elderly being "ripped off" by those who prey on their fears and their desire to feel secure. Chapter 9 will enlighten and enrage all who recognize the need to make older consumers aware of the potential risks when trying some new remedy or sure-fire cure. Yet at the same time, we must keep in mind that older consumers must bare the burden of making themselves aware of products and services in the marketplace.

When considering at-risk elders living alone, the role of the caregiver is vital (chapter 9). The functions they perform and the assistance they provide to family members and loved ones are invaluable. However, while serving the needs of the elderly, these providers of care must also be mindful of their own need to recuperate from the strain of daily responsibilities.

It has been a great joy to work with the group of professionals who have contributed to this volume. They demonstrated a sincere and compassionated understanding of the problems confronting at-risk elders; each has sought to ease the burden of older persons as well as those whose loving concern has inspired them to learn more about how to make life a little better for a generation whose members have given so much.

1

The Uncooperative Elder

Jay Kruse

With people living longer and with the advent of nuclear families, relatives and family members must learn to provide care for our older generation with minimal stress to them and to their families.[1] With 20 percent of the elderly living with relatives, the potential for high levels of stress is heightened for all parties involved.[2] Families frequently go through many changes and challenges that are specific to their elderly members.[3] While caring for the elderly, many difficult situations can arise.[4] Some of the most difficult ones deal with elder refusal to cooperate. Uncooperativeness is a problem with which all caregivers must contend, but it is particularly common in older age groups.[5] Attempts to understand and help a person can be hindered by lack of cooperation.[6] Uncooperative people can be extremely frustrating, especially when efforts are being made to provide assistance.

Uncooperativeness surfaces in many forms. It can range from a passive lack of cooperation to open meanness of character and belligerence. Some of the most common displays of uncooperativeness are poor table manners, lack of hygiene, verbal and physical abuse, refusal to take medication, and refusal to eat or to drink adequate amounts of fluids.[7] When elders fail to cooperate with efforts to help them, conditions can sometimes resemble a psychological wrestling match.[8] From the point of view of the caregiver, this behavior may become tiresome and frustrating. However, every form of uncooperativeness tells us something about the problems that the elder is facing. There is a reason for all behavior, so we need to look at the motivations for uncooperativeness. Lack of cooperation is a clue in itself.[9] The way to deal with uncooperativeness is to treat the factors that cause it. *Loss of independence, mental declines,* and *depression* are perhaps the three most significant causal factors. The more aware we become of the problems that elders face, the more we will understand these causal factors and how they effect the elderly.

LOSS OF INDEPENDENCE

Society does not always love and respect its elders; instead, it tends to place them in dependent roles.[10] This only contributes further to their feelings of inadequacy, hopelessness, loss of self-reliance, and loss of a sense of social value.[11] These feelings trigger the fear and anger that underlie most uncooperative behavior.[12] To the caregiver, this uncooperativeness may appear as willful and foolish obstruction, but to better understand dependence-related uncooperativeness, we need to consider the psychological grounds for such behavior.[13]

Lawrence Breslau and Marie Haug, in their book *Depression and Aging,* offer a unique perspective on the many role changes we experience in life. They start with the premise that old age means dependence. We are a nation of individualists who pride ourselves on our independence. Through childhood and adolescence, growing up means establishing a separate, independent, individual identity, and adulthood is the culmination of this effort. Dependence is not condoned in adulthood, yet society expects its elders to prepare for dependence in later life.

> We come into this world as our parents' children. As we grow up, many of us become parents to our own children. As we grow older still, we become parents to our own parents. Finally, we end up becoming our children's children.[14]

The declining elderly person frequently becomes dependent upon the adult child for food, clothing, shelter, and friendship. In life, we are not prepared to become our parents' parents, or to become our children's children. Breslau and Haug, think it's time we become prepared for these changing roles. We shouldn't infantilize the aged, but we should accept that necessities of life must be provided. Most elderly parents want to live on their own, but near their children. Most value their independence, but as they decline with age they are more likely to live in the same household as their children. These people are then required to accept the help of adult children and bow to their decisions at a time in life when the habits and routines of the older family members have become more fixed then ever before.[15]

Dependence on others is one of the most dreaded role changes associated with old age.[16] It's no wonder there is so much dependent-related uncooperativeness. We need to remember that many of the social roles that are important to elders include many that are crucial at any age and some that acquire particular significance in old age.[17] Some of the neglected social roles include work, sex, leisure pursuits, and the ability to care for ones self.[18] The loss of these important social roles only furthers the sense of hopelessness and decline that often brings about uncooperativeness.[19]

As the motivations for uncooperativeness become clearer, there is a self-fulfilling prophecy that appears. People write off the elderly too often, and don't give them a chance to achieve minimal goals.[20] Families often reward or reinforce the older person for being dependent and for expressions of helplessness. In a sense, then, the older person is rewarded intermittently with attention for *not acting* or for acting out.[21] The blame for being uncooperative is then partially off the shoulders of those who write off the elderly as hopeless.[22] This assumption is frequently transferred to the elderly person, who then *becomes* uncooperative—and why not, since family members give the impression that only belligerent behavior will be given attention?—and the self-fulfilling prophecy is complete.[23]

In order to deal with dependence-related uncooperativeness, we need to put ourselves in the place of the elder person. One way to look at uncooperativeness is as *active resistance,* a defense mechanism employed to preserve self-esteem and ward off invasions.[24] The elderly person may view the conflict of the pleading caregiver as a contest of wills.[25] Uncooperativeness can therefore be seen as a sign of strength, a vain attempt at defiant compensation for real declines in independence and self-reliance.[26] The refusal of older persons to cooperate may be an attempt to control an area—any area—of their lives.[27] Although lack of cooperation or resistance are unpleasant, resistance at least encompasses a livelier concept.[28] A fighting spirit may be healthier than a quiet one.[29] Differing from passive uncooperativeness (which will be discussed later with depression), active resistance is a sign of strength, although misdirected. Active uncooperativeness allows for more focus on the wishes of the elderly person. Therefore, the solution is to honor it, rather than confront it. Attention must be given to the elderly person's needs and lifestyle. All behavior has a reason and in the case of difficult elders it may be very important.[30] Advice and direction should be given when appropriate, with due care taken not to rekindle the fear or anger that caused the uncooperative behavior. Active uncooperativeness calls for wit rather than force: don't try to defeat the elderly person (what purpose would that serve?), but attempt to outwit and win her over, and thus making it *her choice*.[31] It is important to see resistance as a sign of strength and as an attempt to preserve integrity.[32] When the defensive motivations are realized, the role of uncooperative behavior can be dignified. Help can then take the form of teamwork and be mutually rewarding.

In dealing with hesitant or fearful elders, it is important to gain their confidence, not by rushing but by careful listening and showing of sympathy and understanding. The elder's side should be taken, even in disagreement with other relatives, in order to prove your loyalty.[33] To develop or redevelop a healthy relationship is a must.[34] Honoring the elderly's resistance to invasions and joining with them in their desire to remain their own persons may be the best way of securing a helpful relationship.[35] There is a careful balance that should be kept. Personal dignity or rights should never be outweighed or discredited, but at the same time, perspectives and alternatives can be offered.[36] As a caregiver it is possible to give a sort of parental love and permissiveness without violating the person's pride.[37] Even when it seems that the elder is so resistant that nothing will help, he or she can still be bolstered psychologically, even though self-defeating behavior must be overlooked.[38] Overall, when developing a relationship with an uncooperative elder, trust should be created by excepting everything negative, avoiding irritation, and always maintaining one's perspective as a caregiver.[39]

In addition to showing sincere empathy and understanding, the caregiver should also convey a feeling of respect for the elder. Associated with a loss of independence is a feeling of diminished social value and uselessness. Cooperation can sometimes be achieved by showing confidence in the elder's abilities, while at the same time building the person's self-esteem. In a case study where uncooperativeness was attributed to diminished self-esteem and a sense of worthlessness, Robert Gropper came up with an interesting idea. He secured compliance by conveying to the person that he had respect for her intelligence, and gave her a chance to help others at the same time.[40]

CASE STUDY

The client, Mildred, arrived on time for her first appointment. She was unaccompanied as she would be for all subsequent appointments. Immediately after introductions were exchanged an attempt was made to secure a brief history. Mildred then complained that she felt violently ill, perhaps because of a medication interaction. She requested that her appointment be rescheduled because she did not feel able to continue. Because most of the hour was left, I suggested that she lie down for a few minutes in an adjoining room and perhaps we then could try again. Mildred insisted that she must return home immediately or she would become violently ill. This was her first visit; her behavior pattern was not then known to us. She was allowed to leave. An appointment was scheduled for the following week.

Mildred arrived about thirty-five minutes late for her next appointment. The amount of time available for an evaluation was limited. I immediately began the Bender-Gestalt.* After completing the first drawing, she informed me that she had had enough and would not continue. She had not slept the night before because of anxiety about the meeting. She then began to sob loudly and stated that these tests would confirm the fact that she was worthless and, even worse, crazy. She felt that if she continued the tests she would lose her benefits (services from the foundation) and possibly be placed in an institution for the insane.

She believed that her life was totally out of control. She had been taking many tests, both of the physical and mental variety, over the past ten years and nothing improved her condition. She was convinced that this procedure was a total waste of time and we both had "better ways of spending our mornings."

I attempted to explain that the tests were required if she were to continue receiving any services through the foundation. In fact, not completing this evaluation could endanger her benefits. By now our time was up and I once again was forced to reschedule for the following week. Mildred said that she might kill herself before our next Wednesday meeting. I replied that if this came about to have someone inform us so that the time could be assigned to another client. If, however, she was still with us, I definitely expected her the following Wednesday at 11:00 A.M. sharp.

---

*A psychological test used to measure a person's ability to copy a set of geometric designs.

After she left, I searched through her file for some clue that would help me obtain some meaningful cooperation. She seemed to have a history of antagonistic behavior toward professionals. It was obvious that her self-concept was totally diminished. My problem at this point, however, was to reach a meaningful evaluation, not necessarily to improve her self-esteem.

It was apparent that Mildred would not return. She expressed feelings of being helpless, useless, and out of control. But during the week an idea occurred to me. I felt that if I gave her some power along with a sense of value, she might become more cooperative.

It was customary for my secretary to call all clients the day before and remind them of their appointments. In this case, I called Mildred. Before I finished my greeting, Mildred complained about her back, her head, and her general condition of malaise. I decided to give her a chance to improve her self-esteem and perhaps view herself as an individual of worth. If I told her that I was very fond of her and that I really wanted to help her, she would still refuse to meet since she had heard that line many times before. Instead, I shared with her my supposed problem. It was very important to me and the social worker that we finish this evaluation. I explained that we did not have enough data on brighter clients who came to the foundation. The director had informed us that if we did not complete these types of evaluations, our jobs would be in danger. I told Mildred that Susan (the social worker) and I would consider it a personal favor if she would cooperate.

Not only did she appear the next morning on time, but was very cooperative and completed several tests. The following week she returned and completed the remaining tests. During the test-taking there was no indication of any physical complaints. We consistently reiterated to Mildred how much the staff appreciated her cooperation. At the end of the second session, the social worker and I presented Mildred with a small gift as a token of our appreciation. She left beaming.[41]

Although this case study took place in a clinical setting, it is clear that establishing confidence at any level can be a powerful tool. Cooperation was easily achieved by making the client feel intelligent and useful. Self-esteem is an obvious requirement for total health.

Jones and Flickinger state in their essay on therapy for uncooperative patients that we need to dispel the commonly held myth that elders become more and more alienated from their families and die lonely deaths in inhumane institutions.[42] This is wrong. Families tend to provide a lot of support for their elderly members and continue to fulfill this duty throughout the elderly's life. Maintaining hope for the future is a task of paramount importance that all family members can encourage. Meeting this responsibility in preserving a positive attitude can be difficult and draining at times.[43] Eighty percent of all elders have empty expectations for the future and say that they live "day-to-day."[44] For this reason, modern therapy often involves the whole family.[45] It is helpful and indeed essential in some situations if a successful outcome is to occur. Frequently, therapy will help the relatives and caregivers as much as the elderly loved one.[46]

The logical way to deal with dependence-related uncooperativeness is to allow and encourage as much *independence* as possible. Care of the elderly should be aimed at maintenance of maximum possible functional and social independence. Healthcare and social services should be provided in a manner that preserves the dignity of elders and provides an opportunity for personal choice.[47] Many psychologists believe in the "active role," reinforcing the belief that clients have the ability to master the issues in their lives. Elders should be encouraged to continue their independence by actively addressing daily tasks. Frequently, when an elderly person is living independently or alone, complaints of loneliness may lead the family to arrange for their elder to give up independent living and stay with them. Such a move may cause a great deal of stress, and it may not relieve the loneliness that motivated the move.[48]

The elimination of uncooperative behavior requires an integration. First, caregivers must go beyond considering uncooperativeness as a sign of weakness or cowardice in the face of reality.[49] If this stereotype is dropped, many caregivers may find uncooperative patients more heroic than they realized. Once the motivations for this behavior are recognized, caregivers and elders can help to sustain the latter's sense of personal independence.

> It is particularly important to sustain the failing aged patient's sense of personal identity, his intactness as an individual, as his capacities and accustomed resources fade; to assert with him and for him his right to direct his own life; and to bolster his sense of mastery over his own life direction, even in the face of his actual impotence.[50]

SENILITY

Both emotional and mental problems play a role in uncooperative behavior.[51] As the mind deteriorates, the elderly have a decreasing ability to cope with the demands of life. Individuals identified as senile may not be able to communicate their needs to others or to understand what others are trying to communicate to them.[52] Because of this communication barrier, senile elders are seemingly uncooperative.[53] Uncooperative behavior may be seen as an attempt on their part to communicate unmet needs.[54] Failure to understand when confronted with a task or question may result in frustration or combative behavior.[55] All senility-related uncooperativeness seems to arise because of the margin between the elders' altered ability to cope and the demands placed upon them.[56]

Senility-related uncooperativeness occurs in varying degrees and intensities.[57] Episodes can range from the extreme of violence to minor irritability or crying, but they are usually the outcome of an inability to cope with a situation.[58] Features of senility that contribute to uncooperativeness include mood changes, sexual arousal, crying, excessive drinking of fluid, aimless walking, and remoteness or hostility when demands are placed on on effected individual.[59] Minor episodes are usually brief, with verbal expressions of anger or signs of restless tension.[60] This behavior may seem willful when the senile person is being obstinate.[61]

Senile elders are not the only ones who suffer. Sometimes the caregivers get hurt.[62] Uncooperative behavior can be uncontrollable, violent, and potentially harmful to caregivers.[63] Angry patients sometimes hit, punch, bite, and scratch.[64] Disruptive and unexpected behavioral outbursts in senile patients are frightening.[65] Fear and frustration generate anger and hostility, causing the patient to strike out indiscriminately.[66] Family members or caregivers often respond with these same emotions of fear and anger, which only exasperates the situation.[67] Physical abuse to the caregiver results in anxiety over loss of control, and the caregiver becomes frightened and hesitant. The resulting stress creates a less then optimal environment for care.[68] Meddaugh found in her study on abusive elderly, that no abusers possessed clear intellectual functions. The rate of abuse increased with the level of confusion.[69] Abusive elders are frustrated and angry about their confusion and many times are unable to release those feelings through work, exercise, or leisure activities.[70] The confused person may even be clinging to a former way of releasing aggressive tendencies, and confusion prevents finding new outlets for feelings.[71]

To deal with senility-related uncooperativeness, caregivers need to attend to the confusion at the root of the behavior. Some of the resistant behavior of senile elders is marked by extreme anxiety and is thought to be unavoidable and unpredictable.[72] However, much of the behavior can be prevented or modified.[73] These behaviors are more frequent when routines are changed or when the senile person is placed in new surroundings.[74] Even a trip to the doctor or an unfamiliar home can precipitate inappropriate behavior.[75] The best solution is to keep the elder in a balanced and familiar environment as much as possible. Surprises should be avoided. Strange people in the environment may invoke intense fear.[76] Expecting these elders to comply with complex tasks may also precipitate uncooperativeness. Even getting dressed or brushing their teeth are very complex tasks for compromised persons.[77] Resistance to a simple command is one of the signs that it is beyond a person's resources.[78]

Complex tasks can be subdivided into small, manageable components. Plenty of time should be allowed for every task. Attempts to hurry the senile individual will almost certainly increase the potential for intensifying inner tension, perhaps escalating the problematic behavior.[79] Uncooperative behavior is worse when the person is overstimulated or tired.[80] Overall, it is important to remember that senility-related uncooperativeness is not willful obstinate behavior, but a signal that the demands placed on that person exceeds his or her resources. Learning to modify these behaviors is a major goal.[81] This can be achieved by maintaining a familiar environment and a predictable routine. It is important, especially with abusive elders, to pay attention to when they are becoming overwhelmed. They can then be helped to release their feelings in acceptable ways.

DEPRESSION

Although the majority of older people remain productive and happy throughout life, there are still large numbers that suffer from depression.[82] Many of these bouts of depression in turn create episodes of uncooperativeness. Although the factors of uncooperativeness already discussed are also causes of depression, depression-related uncooperativeness is still dealt with as a factor on its own because of its classification as a disease.

Community studies have measured prevalence rates of depression in the elderly (people over age sixty) at from 11 percent to 30 percent.[83] Even more shocking, as many as 25 percent of the reported suicides are people over age sixty-five, even though this age group only represents 10 percent of the population.[84]

Of course varying levels of depression are seen in all age groups, but, unique features contribute to the prevalence of depression in the elderly. Life stresses and changing life situations increase the likelihood of depression occurring in old age. The many losses normally experienced in later life contribute greatly to the high incidence of depression. Bereavement, failing health, loss of social status, retirement, financial insecurities, movement to nursing homes, and the general loss of self-reliance are just a few of the many contributing factors. The mental load is incredible, as 80 percent of the elderly have chronic health problems, 25 percent have limited mobility, 10 percent of men and 25 percent of women are widowed, leaving one out of seven men and one out of three women living alone.[85] Perhaps the greatest trigger in the onset of depression is when two or more of these losses occur at the same time.[86]

Depression is not a well-defined disease, which means neither the caregiver, the spouse, nor the family doctor is likely to diagnose it until it reaches an advanced state.[87] As a society, we are not as willing to treat depression as we are bodily injury.[88] Depression is under-diagnosed, underreported, and undertreated. Less than one-fourth of elderly patients receive the attention they need.

A substantial contributor to the lack of diagnosis is the stereotype we have of the elderly. Many of the symptoms of depression—including physical problems, changes in posture, insomnia, loss of appetite, and failing memory—are all resigned to old age.[89] A distinction between depression and the normal mood of sadness is not always clear.[90] It is also possible for the symptoms to come and go, which makes it even more difficult to diagnose. If depression is not taken care of, however, the consequences can be serious. Those elderly who are effected could accept the down-and-out image of themselves and fail to struggle toward health. Further complicating the diagnosis of depression is its possible appearance as senility, or vice-versa. In some cases it is very difficult to accurately decipher senility and depression. It is important for the caregiver to remember that senility is an over-used term that limits the way we deal with the elderly.[91] Regardless of the reasons, if depression is left untreated, in addition to increasing the level of uncooperativeness, it can be life-threatening.[92]

The types of uncooperativeness that result from depression are different from those caused by the other factors. Depression-related uncooperativeness may appear in two forms: first, the denial of the depression and the refusal to seek treatment, and second, the forms of uncooperativeness that the depression may cause.

Failure to admit depression is very common in the elderly.[93] They are reluctant to ask for help or take advantage of help if it is offered.[94] This denial makes it extremely difficult to get them the help they need. It seems as though there is always stigma attached to mental illness.[95] The mentally ill are viewed as being crazy: elderly people may be worried about their friends or family finding out, thus the treatment of depression may be hindered by fear of talking about the problem. In this situation, the presence of a low-status stranger can help greatly. Sometimes an elder can admit feelings to someone such as a housekeeper with little or no embarrassment.[96]

Very often family members will ultimately suffer from trying to handle problems that are beyond their resources; eventually they realize that professional help is needed.[97] Caregivers should not internalize failure, and should not feel guilty about seeking professional help for loved ones. Although sadness and disappointment can be helped by family love and encouragement, clinical depression requires the assistance of a therapist. In such therapy, family involvement is important in working through the grief experience brought on by the decline of an elder.

Many older patients expect that psychological therapy is only for those who are severely disturbed and that it is used as a prelude to hospitalization. Many think that psychological treatment will not impact on their problems, because it focuses on their attitudes and feelings, which elders may not see as the cause of their problems. Elders often attribute depression to persons or situations in which loss of control plays a key role. Skepticism may be present if a family member has pressured for treatment. The best way to nullify skeptical belief is to present therapy as an educational model, a way to better adjust to this stage of life.[98] What therapy does is offer clients the opportunity to learn about themselves and to learn skills for coping with current and future depression.[99] It is important that the caregiver convey this model to elder patients needing treatment. It may also help to tell them that in therapy, patients do not discuss problems and experience feelings, but that they learn to modify negative thoughts. This will take considerable effort on the part of elders, their therapists, and their families. Everyone works together toward self-reliance. Therapy deals directly with family issues, aiming to develop and maintain interdependence.[100]

The secondary forms of uncooperativeness arising from depression are likely to remain until the depression is treated. The forms of uncooperativeness caused by depression are commonly less aggressive and are more apathetic displays than those of other causal factors. While the anger caused by a loss of independence, or senility, can result in active or passive resistance, depression merely reduces the person's ability to cope.[101] The uncooperative behavior can take a variety of forms: refusal to eat, reluctance to groom oneself, difficulty sleeping, refusal to move about, and social withdrawal. It is as though life no longer seems worth living. Frequently, the depressed elderly will have a total lack of energy. It is difficult for them to deal with the nothingness of depression. At least with anger there is some hope since strength is being shown, even though it is misdirected. Anger and depression exert opposite influences on the elderly.[102] Anger is sometimes used to treat depression-related uncooperativeness in difficult situations. Peterson, in her essay entitled "The Role of Depression and Anger," offers an interesting case study on the use of anger in the treatment for depression, but stresses that it should be used judiciously and only after more conventional therapy has failed.[103] Again, although in a clinical setting, it is a good example of how the uncooperativeness associated with depression and that associated with anger are quite different.

CASE STUDY

The patient, Mr. G., was an eighty-eight-year-old gentleman with congestive heart failure. He had been hospitalized for over two weeks at the time of the referral and his physical disease and his general disinterest in physical therapy, meals, and visits from relatives were due to emotional rather than physical dysfunction. Mr. G. had also been uncooperative with the nursing staff. He was eating poorly and preferred to remain flat on his back despite the frequently voiced concern that pneumonia could develop if he did not spend some portion of his time sitting upright. He refused to get up and move about, demanding a bedside urinal instead, even though he was capable of walking and it was a necessary part of his recovery.

Although Mr. G. explicitly denied being depressed, statements like "I came to the hospital to die, only the doctors won't let me" and "I'm nothing but a burden to my children" were consistent with a diagnosis of depression, as were his sleeping and eating disturbances. Mr. G. was not only uncooperative when it came to eating, walking, and physical therapy, but he was unwilling to be involved in attempts to improve his mood or to reinvolve him with the world. I had tried a wide range of techniques from being sensitive and empathic to being brisk and business-like, but Mr. G. would plead that he was too tired to talk that day, that it was of no use, or that my time would be better spent with the younger patients on the ward who could still look forward to a full life. Mr. G.'s eyesight made reading and television unrewarding, yet he resisted the use of tape-recorded stories and music obtained for him. Even sitting quietly together failed to build rapport. Mr. G. could stare fixedly out of the window for hours on end, refusing to communicate.

One morning a new aide on the ward awakened Mr. G. Not having his false teeth in place, and dazed from sleep, Mr. G. seemed incoherent to the aide who, ignoring his patient's muted protests, lifted him out of bed and into a wheelchair, all the while murmuring what the aide assumed to be consoling reminders of the name of the hospital, the city in which it was located, the current date, and the fact that the linen in the room needed changing and the floor needed to be mopped. In the meantime, Mr. G. would enjoy a nice sit in the hall.

Mr. G. was accustomed to hearing the nursing staff's pleading and cajoling, and my, externally patient and responsive stance. Being unceremoniously dumped into a wheelchair ("I'm not paralyzed, you know. I've still got the use of my legs!"), wheeled out into the public hallway in his hospital gown ("Couldn't have been more than 60 degrees out there and I'm sitting there with my personal parts in the breeze!"), left there for a prolonged period of time ("I must have been there for three hours, with everyone ignoring me"), and, most of all, being spoken to as if he were senile ("Talked to me like I was a baby! Did I know where I was? I sure as hell knew more than that kid did!") enraged Mr. G. Surprisingly, an enraged Mr. G. was apparently a more adaptive individual.

When I came by with my daily "Want to talk about anything?" I was greeted by a new man. Color in his cheeks, fire in his eyes, sitting erect without nursing staff entreaties, he told me about the dreadful way he had been treated. Then he began sliding back toward apathy and hopelessness. On the third day, I again found him lying flat on his back (against medical advice) and "too tired" to talk to me. Taking a deep mental breath, I replied that if he were too exhausted or confused to talk, I could return later when his mind seemed more clear. Instantly, I had a willing conversational partner, ready to testily explain to me that confusion had nothing to do with it. I elevated his bed and we did some good work in the next hour.

In spite of this initially positive impact, I felt the anger could be as problematic as the depression in the long run. Although for the next week it served a useful therapeutic function: I worked furiously to replace it with a more adaptive vehicle. I pointed out that individuals like the aide made mistakes in part because of a lack of knowledge of the elderly and their abilities. There was a lot of educating to be done with most people. Perhaps a handout could be written . . . but by whom? Mr. G.'s failing eyesight did allow him to write in a large wavering script. Following the completion of the project, he wrote a piece on the secrets to a successful forty-year marriage; later he wrote his children about some important family memories. Nursing staff reminders and the availability of a desk with paper down the hall increased his walking. The anger, although sometimes still present, was largely replaced by a new reaction toward feeling useless: Mr. G.'s more typical desire to help others.

Again, because anger is a potentially destructive and dangerous emotion, it should be used sparingly and judiciously as a therapeutic vehicle, and never before trying more conventional techniques. However, as a method of breaking through depression to reach the elderly patient, this technique would seem to have promise.[104]

Unless depression is treated, progress is slow, sluggish, or nonexistent.[105] The caregiver must understand that depression can trigger a total loss of motivation for change.[106] To try would be meaningless as there is a total collapse of self-esteem.[107] The restrictive communication of depressed elders makes it especially difficult: not only does the older person suffer, but so does the caregiver—from the unpredictability of the disease.[108] Depression is episodic in nature and has the tendency to retreat naturally. For long-term well-being, therapy is usually needed. It is unlikely that the elderly can pull out of depression on their own. However, once therapy is started, the potential for favorable and immediate outcome is good. It's a gratifying experience for everyone to see an elder's negative self-image fade as the future quickly brightens.[109]

NOTES

1. D. I. Meddaugh, "Staff Abuse by the Nursing Home Patient," in *The Elderly Uncooperative Patient* (New York: Haworth Press, Inc., 1987).

2. Ibid.

3. S. Jones and M. A. Flickinger, "Contextual Family Therapy for Families with an Impaired Elderly Member: A Case Study," in *The Elderly Uncooperative Patient* (New York: Haworth Press, Inc., 1987).

4. A. C. Walsh, "The Uncooperative Geriatric Patient," in *The Elderly Uncooperative Patient* (New York: Haworth Press, Inc., 1987).

5. G. G. Merill, "Uncooperative Patients," in *The Elderly Uncooperative Patient* (New York: Haworth Press, Inc., 1987).

6. Ibid.

7. R. Bright, "The Use of Music Therapy and Activities with Demented Patients Who Are Deemed 'Difficult to Manage,' " in *The Elderly Uncooperative Patient* (New York: Haworth Press, Inc., 1987).

8. H. T. Burr, "The Patient As Hero: A Psychotherapeutic Approach to Work with Resistant Aged Patients," in *The Elderly Uncooperative Patient* (New York: Haworth Press, Inc., 1987).

9. Merill, "Uncooperative Patients."

10. L. D. Breslau and M. R. Haug, *Depression and Aging* (New York: Springer Publishing Company, 1983).

11. Ibid.

12. Burr, "The Patient As Hero."

13. Ibid.

14. Breslau and Haug, *Depression and Aging.*

15. Ibid.

16. Meddaugh, "Staff Abuse by the Nursing Home Patient."

17. Breslau and Haug, *Depression and Aging.*

18. Ibid.

19. R. Grooper, "Strategic Oneupmanship: A Technique for Managing the Uncooperative Client," in *The Elderly Uncooperative Patient* (New York: Haworth Press, Inc., 1987).

20. Burr, "The Patient As Hero."

21. D. R. Eyde and J. A. Rich, "Psychological Distress in Aging: A Family Management Model," *Journal of Gerontology 31,* no. 3 (1976): 278–82.

22. Burr, "The Patient As Hero."

23. Ibid.

24. Ibid.

25. Ibid.

26. Ibid.

27. W. C. Raber, F. Lamboo, and L. Mitchell-Pederson, "From Duckling to Swan," in *The Elderly Uncooperative Patient* (New York: Haworth Press, Inc., 1987).

28. Burr, "The Patient As Hero."

29. Ibid.

30. Merill, "Uncooperative Patients."

31. Burr, "The Patient As Hero."

32. Ibid.

33. Walsh, "The Uncooperative Geriatric Patient."

34. Raber, Lamboo, and Mitchell-Pederson, "From Duckling to Swan."

35. Burr, "The Patient As Hero."

36. F. Bemak, "Four Step Clinical Intervention Model: Treatment With the Resistant Patient," in *The Elderly Uncooperative Patient* (New York: Haworth Press, Inc., 1987).

37. Burr, "The Patient As Hero."

38. Ibid.

39. Merill, "Uncooperative Patients," and Raber, Lamboo, and Mitchell-Pederson, "From Duckling to Swan."

40. Grooper, "Strategic Oneupmanship: A Technique for Managing the Uncooperative Client."

41. Ibid.

42. Jones and Flickinger, "Contextual Family Therapy for Families with an Impaired Elderly Member."

43. Breslau and Haug, *Depression and Aging.* See also Jones and Flickinger, "Contextual Family Therapy for Families with an Impaired Elderly Member."

44. Breslau and Haug, *Depression and Aging.*

45. G. Kirk, "A Community Mental Health Center's Approach to Handling the Uncooperative Aging Client: 'Team Approach,' " in *The Elderly Uncooperative Patient* (New York: Haworth Press, Inc., 1987).

46. Walsh, "The Uncooperative Geriatric Patient."

47. G. Lesnoff-Carauglia, *Health Care of the Elderly: Strategies for Prevention and Intervention* (New York: Human Science Press, 1980).

48. Breslau and Haug, *Depression and Aging.*

49. Burr, "The Patient As Hero."

50. Ibid.

51. Ibid.

52. Ibid.

53. L. French, "Uncooperativeness as a Latent Indicator of Dementia among the Mentally Retarded," in *The Elderly Uncooperative Patient* (New York: Haworth Press, Inc., 1987).

54. L. P. Gwyth and M. Blazer, "Family Therapy and the Dementia Patient," *American Family Physician, 3* (1984): 149–56.

55. M. A. Bartol, "Nonverbal Communication in Patients with Alzheimer's Disease," *Journal of Gerontological Nursing 5,* no 4 (1979): 21–31.

56. J. M. Thornbury, "Catastrophic Reactions," in *The Elderly Uncooperative Patient* (New York: Haworth Press, Inc., 1987).

57. Ibid.

58. K. Goldstein, "The Effect of Brain Damage on the Personality," *Psychiatry 4* (1979): 21–31.

59. French, "Uncooperativeness as a Latent Indicator of Dementia among the Mentally Retarded."

60. Goldstein, "The Effect of Brain Damage on the Personality."

61. N. L. Mace and P. V. Rabins, *The 36-Hour Day* (Baltimore: Johns Hopkins Press, 1981).

62. Meddaugh, "Staff Abuse by the Nursing Home Patient."

63. Thornbury, "Catastrophic Reactions."

64. Ibid.

65. Ibid.

66. Ibid.

67. Bartol, "Nonverbal Communication in Patients with Alzheimer's Disease."

68. Meddaugh, "Staff Abuse by the Nursing Home Patient."

69. Ibid.

70. Ibid.

71. Ibid.

72. Mace and Rabins, *The 36-Hour Day.*

73. Ibid.

74. Thornbury, "Catastrophic Reactions."

75. Ibid.

76. Ibid.

77. Ibid.

78. Ibid.

79. Goldstein, "The Effect of Brain Damage on the Personality."

80. Bartol, "Nonverbal Communication in Patients with Alzheimer's Disease."

81. Thornbury, "Catastrophic Reactions."

82. Breslau and Haug, *Depression and Aging.*

83. S. Meeks and S. A. Murrell, "Depressive Symptoms in Older Adults: Predispositions, Resources, and Life Experiences," in *Annual Review of Gerontology and Geriatrics, 11* (New York: Springer Publishing Company, Inc., 1992).

84. H. S. Resnik and J. M. Cantor, "Suicide and Aging," *Journal of the American Geriatrics Society 18* (1970): 1152–58.

85. A. Raskin and G. Sathananthan, "Depression in the Elderly," *Psychopharmacology Bulletin 15,* no. 2 (1979): 14–16.

86. E. Bibring, "Psychoanalysis and Dynamic Psychotherapies," *Journal of the American Psychoanalytic Association 2,* no. 4 (1954): 745–70.

87. A. Horowitz, "Social Network and Pathways into Psychiatric Treatment," *Social Forces 56,* no. 1 (1977): 86–105.

88. Breslau and Haug, *Depression and Aging.*

89. L. J. Epstein, "Symposium on Age Differentiation in Depressive Illness," *Journal of Gerontology, 31,* no. 3 (1976): 278–82.

90. Breslau and Haug, *Depression and Aging.*

91. Thornbury, "Catastrophic Reactions."

92. Breslau and Haug, *Depression and Aging.*

93. Ibid.

94. G. E. Shute, "Psychotherapy of Reluctant, Depressed Elders," in *The Elderly Uncooperative Patient* (New York: Haworth Press, Inc., 1987).

95. Breslau and Haug, *Depression and Aging.*

96. Ibid.

97. Horowitz, "Social Network and Pathways into Psychiatric Treatment."

98. Shute, "Psychotherapy of Reluctant, Depressed Elders."

99. Ibid.

100. Jones and Flickinger, "Contextual Family Therapy for Families with an Impaired Elderly Member."

101. L. Peterson, "Rx: Anger," in *The Elderly Uncooperative Patient* (New York: Haworth Press, Inc., 1987).

102. Ibid.

103. Ibid.
104. Ibid.
105. Ibid.
106. Ibid.
107. Bibring, "Psychoanalysis and Dynamic Psychotherapies."
108. Breslau and Haug, *Depression and Aging.*
109. Eyde and Rich, "Psychological Distress in Aging."

ADDITIONAL REFERENCES

Salzman, C., and R. I. Shader. "Clinical Evaluation of Depression in the Elderly," in *Psychiatric Symptoms and Cognitive Loss in the Elderly: Evaluation and Assessment Techniques.* Washington, D.C.: Hemisphere. 1979.

Soldo, B. J. "America's Elderly in the 1980s," *Population Bulletin, 35,* no. 4 (1980). Washington D.C.: Population Reference Bureau, Inc.

2

Drug Misuse among the Elderly

James R. Beal

If you were to ask someone on the street on any given day who he or she thought the typical drug abuser/misuser was, the reply may be something along the lines of a teenager from the "wrong side of the tracks." Unfortunately, this is the stereotypical view shared by most people because it is the one receiving the most publicity in the media. There exists in the United States, however, a much more subtle and unknown type of drug abuse and misuse. It does not involve teenagers or college students or gang members of any type; it involves our own elderly population.

There are a number of reasons why elders would be in the position of misusing or abusing drugs. In many cases elders may not understand exactly what drug it is that is being taken, and, therefore, they are naive to the nature of the reactions they have to the drug. In other instances, the drug, often a common painkiller or medication, provides a form of escape or denial from the problems of life.

These two situations vary in that one is physical, while the other is physiological and also emotional. Understanding the nature and various characteristics of misuse and abuse of drugs by the elderly is paramount if a loved one is to be prevented from falling into such a trap, or, if it is too late for prevention, for successful rehabilitation out of a dependence situation.

Before much thought can be given to prevention or rehabilitation, however, steps must be taken to understand

- the types of drugs, their effects and dangers;

- the causes of misuse or abuse of drugs;

- the signals of dependence or misuse by an elder;

- the role of proper education and openness in preventing dependence or abusive situations; and

- the methods of handling misuse, in addition to education.

Here we will cover the above information in addition to providing some typical scenarios or cases. Following the cases will be an application of the information to the particular case, thereby mapping a solution to the problem.

After reading this chapter it is hoped that family members, caregivers, and interested parties will be better prepared to deal with a drug misuse or abuse situation when confronting an elder who has chosen to remain in the community as opposed to entering a supervised care program (e.g., a nursing home or managed-care facility). Being unsupervised, elders are subject to a number of risks, both obvious and obscure. For this reason, responsible intervention may be needed on the part of the caregiver, not to usurp the sovereignty of the elder, but to facilitate a lasting solution to a potentially catastrophic problem.

The worst part of the problem is that in most cases, the elders misuse drugs out of lack of proper or complete knowledge of the medication regimen due to miscommunication with or failure to understand the physician, as opposed to open or blatant abuse. Especially in these cases, elders need a caring and informed person to intervene, whether they know it or not.

RATIONALE FOR INTERVENING: DEFINING THE PROBLEM

More often than not, an elder is misusing a drug or medication as opposed to abusing it. Misuse can largely be attributed to noncompliance on the part of the elder due to lack of knowledge of the medication regimen (dosage, frequency, and the duration that the medicine is prescribed for). On the other hand, in situations of abuse the elder has at least some knowledge of using the drug, though the person may deny that the drug is being abused. Frequently abused drugs include over-the-counter (OTC) and prescription medications as well as alcohol, tobacco, and even controlled substances (i.e., narcotics, marijuana, etc.).

Although the abuse of controlled substances is an extremely serious problem no matter who is involved, including elders, it will be, for the most part, excluded from this discussion. Only a very small fraction of the elderly population is expected to use these substances, and, at this mature age, the use is probably very well hidden. Nonetheless, some attention will be paid at least to signals of possible abuse and available resources. Here emphasis will be given mainly to OTC and prescription drug misuse and abuse.

When elders choose to remain at home in the community and not enter some type of supervised care program, they give up the security of supervision for the comfort of home. The familiarity of home surroundings can not only be therapeutic in the treatment of many psychological and mild physical ailments, but also it can make the final years of life happier, easier, and more enjoyable. Unfortunately, remaining at home unsupervised also means that some risks are being taken, especially in light of the fact that as the human body and mind mature, physical and mental capacities can be adversely affected.

As the body deteriorates slowly with age, it is more susceptible to illness and fluctuations in health. The miracles of modern medicine, however, enable us in many cases to relieve painful or uncomfortable symptoms of bodily ailments. However, the body's reaction to these miracle drugs changes over time, as it weakens with age.[1] Compound this with the fact that of all the people in American society, the aged population (those sixty-five years of age and older) consume more medication per capita than any other segment of society,[2] and potential problems become evident. What makes this problem even more pronounced is that an average elder may take three, five, or more *different* medications every day!

The plethora of medications both available to and required by elders is enough to confuse the sharpest of minds. What makes the problem especially dizzying for many elders is that not only do they not understand what all the medications are that they are taking, but too often they do not even know exactly why they are taking them. Couple this with the reality that elders often are losing some of their mental faculties as they grow older, and it becomes clear that the potential for noncompliance with the drug regimen, whether intentional or unintentional, increases greatly with age.

Noncompliance with—in essence, misusing—the proper medication schedule can have some very grave consequences for elders, families, and caregivers. Physical manifestations of medication misuse include possible drug-to-drug reactions due to either taking the wrong drugs, consuming the wrong dosages, or both; potential drug-to-lifestyle reactions where the elder is unaware of the harmful effects of improperly combining a medication with some aspect of his or her daily life (e.g., eating a certain food, exposure to sun, etc.); and the altered presentation of an illness, where the illness may appear as something it isn't due to improper dosages of medication.[3] In the last case, a physician may mistake the reaction to misused drug(s) as a new symptom and prescribe an additional medication in response, thereby increasing both the possibility of future health problems and the monthly medicine bill.

Other consequences of drug misuse include addiction, whether psychological, physiological, emotional, or social. The last thing in the world an elder needs is to be dependent on a drug that isn't helping to maintain or improve health, or may even be hindering the person's health and is costing probably significant amounts of money over several months. The economic aspects of drug misuse or abuse, though small compared to the necessity of continued good or improved health on the part of the elder, can loom large in an elder's life, especially if a precarious financial situation exists (as is the case with too many elders in the United States) and the medication being misused is doing more harm than good.

The problems related to drug misuse or abuse among the elderly are many. Whether it's the threat of deteriorating health due to poor administration of medications or the increased financial burden when an elder takes too much or too many different types of the wrong medicine, situations of misuse must be corrected, either by educating elders to take charge of the drug regimen or by intervening.

CASE STUDY

After a series of complicated surgeries, John was recovering reasonably well. His doctor had him on a moderate exercise plan, a good diet, and a battery of medications. Some of his medication was for his heart— John had had a triple bypass performed a while ago—including an anticoagulative agent, a cardiovascular dilating agent (two cardiac drugs aimed at the treatment of heart disease) and an anti-infection agent.[4] His doctor had also put John on some vitamin supplements. All in all, John was supposed to take a total of nine pills of various types each day at different times.

All John knew was that he was taking "vitamins and heart pills"; his doctor had tried to explain the nature of the medications, but was unable to communicate this information in language that John could understand. As a result, John often neglected to take some pills, (a) because he didn't understand what the drugs did and often felt fine without them, and (b) because he did not have any sort of organizational system to aid him in remembering what to take, when, and in what dosages. Not only was John wasting money by not taking all of the medication he was buying (his medication bill totalled about $300 each month), but also he was endangering his health by taking less medication, thereby misusing the drugs that he should have been consuming regularly.

Situation

John, a sixty-nine-year-old living at home, isn't adhering to his medication regimen. This noncompliance is due to a general lack of understanding of the drugs he has been instructed to take.

Threats

By continuing to disregard his medication instructions, John is risking serious medical consequences aggravated by sporadic drug treatment. The distress arising from irregular drug exposure is increasing John's chance of acquiring an infection as a result of a weakened immune system from this stress; in addition, he risks aggravating his present medical situation.[5]

TYPES OF DRUGS USED BY THE ELDERLY

As earlier stated, seniors account for more per capita drug consumption, both over-the-counter and prescription drugs, than any other segment of the population. In fact, in 1975, when the elderly (sixty-five years of age and older) made up only 11 percent of the population, they consumed over 25 percent of all drugs.[6] Today, as our society gradually ages due to advances in medical technology and increased standard of living, this segment of the population continues to grow. As this happens, it will be more and more important to ensure, on an individual level, that the drugs being consumed by elders are purposeful and effective. Anything else is a waste of money and health.

There are several reasons why the elderly are the biggest consumers of drugs in the United States. First, and most obvious, is that elders are more susceptible to bodily ailments than any other age group.[7] In addition, older persons tend to experience chronic problems, where the drug acts as a treatment but for the most part relieves pain and suffering.

One factor skewing the actual percentage of drug consumption by the elderly may have been the large-scale mismanagement and mis-administration of medication in extended care institutions, the same phenomenon that has in recent times supported the broad-based move toward deinstitutionalization. Nonetheless, the elderly are significant consumers of drugs for a variety of reasons, but mainly because the human body tends to deteriorate with age, increasing the likelihood of bodily affliction and ailment.

Several questions, then, must be addressed: What are the major types of medications and drugs used by the elderly? For what purpose(s) are they used? How do we know if they are necessary?

There are a number of categories of drugs, and in each category may be thousands of different drugs, each under a different name—a trade name—depending upon the company that makes it. Often-times, it is impossible to tell what the drug is or what it does simply by looking at its name. This is another reason why good physician-patient relationships are necessary to understanding the nature of any prescribed medication regimen. At least an approximate knowledge of the function and nature of a drug is essential if we are to ensure that the drug does not become misused.

Below are listed some of the most common types of drugs used by elders along with their basic functions. They are listed in order of prevalence as established by a study of over 1,700 elders in Dunedin, Florida.[8]

Anti-hypertensive Agents

These drugs are used to lower and/or combat the effects of high blood pressure. They either slow down the heart by a small proportion or they make the contractions of the heart somewhat smaller. Either of these has the effect of decreasing blood flow, thus lowering blood pressure. In some cases the drug will act to dilate (open) the blood vessels in the periphery of the body (arms, legs) so that the blood has more area in which to flow, which also lowers overall blood pressure. High blood pressure is bad because it increases the chances of an aneurysm (popped blood vessel) in addition to making the heart work too hard. Nearly 31 percent of elders surveyed in the Dunedin study were taking some type of anti-hypertensive agent.[9]

Vitamins

Proper daily allowances of vitamins are important to any person, but to the elderly, who have a higher susceptibility to ailment and affliction, it is especially important. Careful use of vitamin supplements can help the body prepare to fight off disease, as well as increase and maintain good general health.

Cardiac Drugs

These drugs are used primarily in the treatment of various forms of heart disease. They may perform the functions of heart rate regulation, heart muscle stimulation or relaxation, or heart blood flow equalization. In the Dunedin study, nearly 15.5 percent of all elders used some type of cardiac drug.[10]

Cardiovascular Dilators

Cardiovascular dilators do just that; they dilate (open) the vasculature (arteries and veins) of the cardiac blood systems (blood flow to the heart). These drugs open up the blood vessels that supply the heart, ensuring a constant and adequate supply of blood, which, of course, is necessary to the heart's proper function. A typical elder using these drugs may be (or may have been) a candidate for bypass surgery or some type of angioplasty (cleaning, opening, or stretching a blood vessel to let the blood flow more easily). Roughly 13 percent of elders in the Florida study were using a cardiovascular dilator.[11]

Laxatives

Laxatives are drugs that affect the G.I. (gastro-intestinal) system. They either act to make the feces softer and easier to pass through the bowels, or they relax and contract the bowel muscles to induce defecation. However they work, laxatives regulate the body's waste disposal system. Irregularity can cause a number of problems in addition to great discomfort and an increased risk of developing colon cancer. A good diet can sometimes, but not always, take the place of an over-the-counter or prescribed laxative.

Tranquilizers

These drugs act to calm the body's systems, generally decreasing the stressful loads placed upon them. Although very relaxing, tranquilizers are different from sedatives in that their only form of pain relief lies in the fact that they are especially useful if the pain is caused by muscle contraction. In the Dunedin study, only 8.7 percent of all elders surveyed were on some type of tranquilizer prescription.[12]

In addition to these categories of drugs, elders recovering from recent surgery may be prescribed an anti-infection drug, an anti-rejection drug (in the case of transplants or a surgery where an object foreign to the host body has been implanted), an immunostimulant (a drug stimulating an immune response), or a drug in some way related to disease treatment (e.g., chemotherapy for cancer or a specific drug for AIDS).

The Dunedin study notes that the above list of drugs was typical of noninstitutionalized elders who were randomly selected for hypertension screenings. The medications used in extended care facilities or institutions varied from the above list to include analgesics, sedative-hypnotic drugs, as well as a marked increase in the use of laxatives and tranquilizers. The Dunedin study, though conducted in the late 1970s, was nevertheless cited in a National Institute of Drug Abuse publication in 1983, which, I trust, does not make this information too obsolete. In fact, information on drug misuse or abuse among the elderly is usually difficult to find and sparse even when found.

To actually learn about the physical or psychological symptoms that appear when a drug is used properly or misused, you may read any of a number of medication resources currently on the market. Because there are so many different types and variations of drugs, it would be impossible to describe each drug separately and its effects in any format smaller than a large book or reference volume. Consequently, in addition to honest and open communication with a physician, an elder—or at least the caregiver—might choose to obtain a copy of some type of guide to medication. They are located in almost any library or bookstore under the category of "medicine" or "health."

WHY AND WHEN DRUGS ARE MISUSED

Sources usually categorize the reasons for drug misuse as lack of knowledge or noncompliance on the part of the elder. This noncompliance or lack of education is largely due to a poor, or at least noncommunicative, relationship between elders and physicians. This is caused when the physician either does not fully explain the reasoning behind a medication regimen or does not ensure that the elder actually understands what is said, even after the elder *claims* to understand.

Unfortunately, it is a significant factor of human nature not to admit lack of knowledge about a subject, even when this action can be detrimental to the one's health. This type of defense mechanism, though perhaps useful when trying to get a pesky salesman off your back at a retail store, is not, however, a good idea when listening to a doctor describe the state of your health and the rationale behind a recommended treatment.

Physicians have the responsibility to describe the reasons for their diagnoses and how they intend to develop a treatment plan. In reality, this does not always happen, because it is not so simple a task. In the event that an elder has a physicain who is relatively unwilling to justify a prescription, either a new physician or outside information could be sought. Although finding a new doctor may not be possible, there exist many outside sources of information on drugs and medications available to consumers. Understanding the nature and content of the medication regimen prescribed to an elder is the first step in identifying any potential misuse.

All in all, an elder is less likely to adhere to a medication schedule when little information is disclosed about the medicine. Indeed, the older person may rationalize that if she feels well, why should the medication be continued, especially when it is often expensive and has unpleasant side effects? This is the main attitude behind drug misuse, which, often as not, is intentional.

Drug misuse itself can take many forms. Patients can underuse, overuse, and misuse medication. Underuse occurs when the elder does not administer a complete dosage with the frequency recommended by the physician. A sign of underuse is a bottle containing some prescription but where the period of the prescription on the bottle has expired, indicating that the pills were either not taken in a timely fashion or not consumed in the specified quantity.

Overuse occurs when the patient finishes the prescription in advance due to an accelerated rate of drug intake. For example, the elder would take six tablets a day instead of the prescribed four. ("Besides, if four work well enough, then six will make me feel that much better!") This usually occurs when the drug provides particular relief from the symptoms of an ailment—e.g., a pain relief agent for an arthritis sufferer. This excessive use of one or more drugs is especially serious, as the potential side effects are heightened with this type of overdose, however mild it may be, and adverse reactions with other medications, food, or lifestyle may be induced.

Drug misuse usually entails either over- or underuse and/or another type of improper adherence to the specifications of the prescription. For instance, certain types of drugs are most effective or possibly only effective at certain times of the day or under specific physical conditions. Consuming dairy products when directed not to do so or taking a specific drug at the wrong time would be examples of drug misuse.

IDENTIFYING DRUG MISUSE: CLUES AND SIGNALS

There are several telltale signs of potential drug misuse or abuse, particularly when dealing with an elder. A general lack of organization of medications (a jumble of bottles, collections of similar—though different—pills) is one such indicator of possible misuse. Figure 1 lists some common signs of potential medication misuse.

Figure 1

SIGNS OF POTENTIAL DRUG MISUSE

- Disorganized medicine cabinet, a jumble of bottles

- Bottles with labels missing

- Medications showing expired prescriptions

- Clusters of bottles, pills, liquids, or other medications, all of which are difficult to distinguish

- The lack of a medication calendar or some other type of organizational device, especially when a large number of medications is involved

- A lack of understanding on the part of the elder as to exactly what is to be taken

- The appearance that the elder may be taking the medication at irregular, unprescribed intervals

- The tendency for an elder to reach for a pill or a bottle of medication when experiencing an uncomfortable symptom as opposed to checking to see if the time is appropriate for the next scheduled dosage— assuming, of course, that the drug is not of the type to warrant such an action (e.g., nitroglycerine in the event of heartrate irregularity, bronchial mist at the time of an asthma attack, etc.)

- An obvious or apparent adverse reaction to a drug or medication (e.g., disorientation, unusual forgetfulness, vomiting, etc.)

- Mixing incompatible drugs (Consulting a physician or pharmacist, or a drug and medication handbook will help determine if this is likely.)

- Signs of dependence, including paranoia at not being near to the drug or not having the medication available, or undue relief at taking the medication (possible psychological dependence)

It is especially important for the caregiver to supervise the medication regimen for the elder, even if it is in a silent manner, to prevent serious or otherwise adverse reactions from taking place.

CASE STUDY

Margaret suffers from relatively severe arthritis. Her physician has prescribed an anti-inflammatory agent as well as a pain-killer. Even with this medication, she finds it difficult to perform even the most basic daily chores, such as dressing herself or making a meal, but at least the pain is lessened. Sometimes the pain is so bad that she can hardly bear it.

She hadn't seen her doctor for almost a year; it always seemed like such a hassle arranging a ride downtown, where the doctor kept her practice. The prescription given to Margaret was renewable, but when it was given, it was under the assumption that she would be stopping in for regular checkups. Margaret continued to have the pharmacy send her the pain-killers, feeling their soothing effects, while neglecting the anti-inflammatory agent. Whenever she felt the sharp, aching pains return to her hands and joints, she would reach for the bottle of pills and pop one or two into her mouth.

Situation

Margaret has a serious problem. She is misusing her medications, which are meant to work together. This is due in large part to the fact that she does not completely understand the nature of her medication.

Threats

In addition, by not seeing her physician regularly, Margaret is perpetuating an already very uncomfortable condition, a problem that may be relieved by a change in medication or by a consistent application of her current prescription.

ADDRESSING THE PROBLEM

Recognizing that the abuse or misuse of medication is occurring is the most difficult element in solving the larger problem, namely, prevention. Drugs are most effective when used properly, and elders must be made to understand this and to comply with the proper prescription. If an elder fails to adhere to prescriptions, intervention may be necessary.

Intervening in someone's affairs is not always an easy task. Caution must be used when doing so, especially in the case of an elder who has chosen to remain at home and not to enter a care program. There is a strong possibility that the older person will be very protective of his or her privacy, and improper intervention could be very destructive to the relationship between the elder and the caregiver. Trust must be maintained if a lasting solution is to be reached.

In the event that a gentle and caring approach to providing assistance to the elder is not effective, information on dealing with uncooperative patients can be found in chapter 1 of this book. However, once the way has been cleared for intervention, there are many effective methods of dealing with the problems of drug misuse.

Recognizing that lack of education is a major factor in noncompliance or misuse, steps should first be taken to improve the elder's understanding of the medication. For best results, use terms that are readily understood. Figure 2 gives several examples of possible explanations for the various drugs and their uses.

Figure 2

EXPLAINING MEDICATIONS IN LAY TERMS

Anti-hypertensive Agents

These agents prevent the heart from working too hard and putting too much pressure on blood vessels. They are used in conditions where blood vessels, which are normally stretchy, like a balloon, don't stretch very well. It's like filling a balloon with water: if too much water is put into the balloon and the rubber does not stretch, it may break. Similarly, if blood vessels break, doctors might have some problems fixing the leak.

Cardiac drugs

Cardiac medications are meant to help the heart. (*Cardio* is a Latin term meaning "having to do with the heart.") Sometimes the heart appears to march to its own beat, which would be fine if other body parts didn't need a regular supply of blood to stay healthy. When it feels like your heart is jumping around a little bit—not paying attention to its work—you should take one of these little pills labeled "HEART." They help your heart to relax and to take it easy on the rest of your body for a while.

Analgesics

Analgesics are pain-killers. When part of the body hurts, little sensors called nerves tell the brain that you are feeling pain. Analgesics—your yellow pills labeled "PAIN"—stop your nerves from screaming "PAIN" so loudly. They put a sock in the nerves' mouths. The pain is still there but your brain no longer hears your nerves crying so much.

These are a few examples and, yes, they may even seem a bit silly, but they describe a medication in simple terms. After several times of repeating one or more of these explanations, even the most hardheaded elders (barring those with memory deficiencies) should be able to relate a drug to an effect. Teaching elders about the medications they are taking is half the battle in preventing abuse and misuse.

Unfortunately, many physicians may not have either the time or the patience to sit down with every older person to ensure that a prescribed treatment is completely understood. So often, elders maintain that they understand how to administer a medication, when in fact the opposite is true. It cannot be overstressed that *the actual responsibility for conveying understanding falls on the elder.* Only the patient knows when he or she is clearly aware of what a prescribed drug is and how to take it.

Coming up with simple, understandable examples may not be easy, but with a little perserverance, it can be done. Get hold of a medication handbook, read about the drug, and try to think of a story that relates the drug's function to something the elder would understand (e.g., football, knitting, fishing). Practice first to make sure that the actual conversation with the elder is smooth and fluid and that questions can be answered. Have fun if necessary, but keep in mind that this is still *a very serious matter.*

If the caregiver's help is needed in understanding medications and their functions, and if a drug handbook can't clear things up, possible alternative resources include local pharmacies, clinics, hospitals, and libraries, even poison control hotlines. However it is done, steps must be taken to ensure that elders understand the medications they take if we are to minimize the chance of noncompliance due to lack of knowledge.

In other cases, a prescription may be so complex that even an educated patient has difficulty in keeping the various drugs organized. The following case study illustrates such an example.

CASE STUDY

Richard is recovering from open heart surgery, which took place three months ago. Although his recovery is proceeding nicely, some aggravation has recently surfaced. It is likely due to a lack of adherence to the stringent medication regimen necessary after such a procedure. Richard must take six medications every day.

Some medications thin the blood, others regulate blood pressure, but all have a purpose. Unfortunately though, the medications are intended to be taken at what seems to Richard like random intervals during the day: some in the morning, some at bedtime, some several times during the day. Richard is not very organized nor is he inclined to remembering lots of facts, although he does understand the basic purposes of his medications. Lately, however, he has become more and more frustrated as the confusing schedule for taking his prescribed medications still does not make sense to him.

His physician had suggested that he create a medication calendar, but Richard had long since forgotten this option. Fortunately, his caregiver hadn't. His sister, who also took several medications daily, saw Richard's situation and, knowing Richard's inclination to forget things, helped him to devise a type of calendar system to organize all of his prescriptions.

The system employed the use of an alarm clock (a small one that emitted only pleasant, but noticeable beeps), and an empty ice tray having three rows of eight molds. While one column of three was left empty, the rest served as organizers for the seven days of the week, the three receptacles each serving as a time of the day: morning, midday, or night.

By spending about thirty minutes devising a plan of organization, Richard and his sister (it's important for *both* of them to do it to encourage mutual understanding) were able to make the medication regimen not only easy to understand, but simple to use.

Situation

Richard was in the situation of basically understanding his medications, but being confused by their applications. His recovery was subsequently being hampered.

Threats

Aside from hampering his recovery, misuse of the prescribed drugs could also result in potentially serious consequences, including completely ineffective drug treatments due to misapplication.

Physical methods of organization include calendars of various types: color codes, big lettering, or other easily recognizable media are desirable in constructing some type of medication calendar. The calendar should be easy to build, easy to understand, and easy to maintain (refill). *Once it has been made, a quick call to the physician or pharmacist to verify its accuracy is always a good idea.*

Looking at professionally recommended calendars, such as those already developed by clinics, pharmacies, or physicians is desirable before choosing or making a personal calendar. One strong benefit of a calendar, aside from organizing medication, is that it keeps the responsibility for drug use in the hands of the elder, thus ensuring personal autonomy.

In some cases, regular intervention may still be needed to make certain that the prescription is adhered to regularly. Supervisory steps include regular visits, phone calls, or even arranged visits (e.g., by a neighbor, a friend, or a nurse).

Figure 3 details the physical steps, beyond education, that can be used to prevent drug misuse by an elder.

Figure 3

PREVENTING MISUSE (PHYSICAL METHODS)

- Develop a medication calendar.

- Intervene when necessary, checking regularly for adherence to the prescription.

- Know where and how to find outside help when it's needed (some elders can be very uncooperative).

Drug misuse among America's elderly population is far too common to believe that it cannot happen to your own loved one, a good friend or neighbor, or to the person to whom you are providing care. Fortunately, steps can be taken to alleviate drug misuse or at least minimize its presence. Carefully planned intervention using practical and effective techniques can protect an elder from potential misuse. Since in most instances an elder is misusing a drug or prescription only because he or she lacks complete understanding of its importance, dosage, and times of administration, intervention is particularly valuable: most people, elders included, do not want to intentionally jeopardize their own health. All they need is a loving, caring hand to guide them.

NOTES

1. W. E. Hale, R. G. Marks, and R. B. Stewart. "Drug Use in a Geriatric Population," *Journal of the American Geriatrics Society* 27, no. 8 (1979): 374–44.

2. P. R. Raffoul, J. K. Cooper, and D. W. Love. "Drug Misuse in Older People," *The Gerontologist* 21, no. 2 (1981): 146–50.

3. Marjorie Bogaert-Tullis. "A Resource Guide for Drug Management for Older Persons," (San Francisco: Aging Policy Health Center, 1985), U.S. Department of Health and Human Services.

4. Hale et al., "Drug Use in a Geriatric Population."

5. Ibid.

6. Ibid.

7. Raffoul et al., "Drug Misuse in Older People."

8. Hale et al., "Drug Use in a Geriatric Population."

9. Ibid.

10. Ibid.

11. Ibid.

12. Ibid.

ADDITIONAL REFERENCES

Allee, John Gage (ed.), *Webster's Encyclopedia of Dictionaries: Medical Dictionary.* Ottenheimer Publishers, 1981.

Barnhart, Mary Ann. "The Noncompliant Elderly," in Gerald A. Larue and Rich Bayly's (eds.) *Long-Term Care in an Aging Society.* Buffalo, New York: Prometheus Books, 1991, 119–26.

"Drug Misuse Among the Elderly and Its Impact on Community-Based Care," Hearing transcript: Select Committee on Aging, U.S. House of Representatives, Comm. Pub. No. 101–78, April 19, 1989.

Glantz, M. D. D. M. Peterson, F. J. Whittington (eds.). *Drugs and the Elderly Adult,* National Institute on Drug Abuse, U.S. Department of Health and Human Services, 1983.

Guttman, D. "Patterns of Legal Drug Use by Older Americans," *Addictive Diseases: An International Journal* 3, no. 3 (1978): 337–56.

Zawadski, R. T., G. B. Glazer, E. Lurie. "Psychotropic Drug Use Among Institutionalized and Noninstitutionalized Medicaid Aged in California," *Journal of Gerontology* 33, no. 6 (1978): 825–34.

3

Financial Considerations for Elders on Their Own

James R. Beal

Harvey Jones is seventy years old. Almost one year ago his wife, Ethel, passed away. Throughout their forty-five years of marriage, it was she who had the responsibility of taking care of the home, which included keeping on top of financial matters. They had lived comfortably since Harvey had put in thirty good years as the postmaster at the local post office. His pension, along with their combined social security checks, provided them with enough money to enjoy their retirement. In addition, Ethel's spend-thriftiness—Harvey lovingly called her "his penny-pinching, fun-spoiling gift from who-knows-where"—had ensured them a tidy savings. In her truly loving style, she had made certain that, should anything happen to her, Harvey would be financially secure. She had always considered him "a little loopy, though kind of cute."

With Ethel gone Harvey was forced to take charge of his own financial matters, about which he knew very little. It had taken him two months to find where his wife had kept the checkbook. It seemed to him as though everybody wanted money for some reason. Though he would probably never openly admit it, Harvey is completely lost and confused in this new, somewhat foreign situation.

Harvey had been seeing his doctor for the past several years about his heart, and his neighbors and family had noticed that he seemed a little more forgetful lately. His family—two sons, their wives, and five grandchildren—were very concerned, but lived several hundred miles away and could not keep constant tabs on him. Harvey and Ethel had always been close to the neighbors, but now Harvey seemed to retreat into his home after his wife's death. After many months of futile invitations to go golfing, to see a ball game, or to have dinner, his neighbors gradually gave up trying to keep Harvey involved. Harvey just didn't feel like doing much of anything any more.

Harvey was also getting into trouble, without his knowledge. He frequently overlooked or ignored many financial matters that his wife had handled for the two of them. Health insurance claims and bills, Medicare paperwork, investment documents, and other important papers and letters lay piled up on top of the old desk near the phone in the living room, unopened and unread. Without some intervention by an honest, caring party—welcome or not—Harvey's retirement may not remain so comfortable.

When confronted by his family, Harvey was asked to choose where he would like to live now that his wife was gone and he needed some help. He replied that he would like to remain at home, the home he and his wife had built thirty years before.

INTRODUCTION

For many people there comes a time when a physical or mental disability forces them to choose between a life in a healthcare facility or remaining in their communities in familiar surroundings. Their condition is not serious enough to require admission to a permanent care facility, but they must take steps to maintain their personal security. Both of the above choices have their positive and negative aspects.

Healthcare facilities usually offer access to professionals skilled in their fields who have the latest life-saving equipment at their disposal. Some people question the quality of life, however, when an individual is faced with an existence almost totally lacking in personal familiarity and comfort. In some cases, this can be more debilitating than a physical affliction. Personal familiarity can be maintained, however, if the individual chooses to remain at home in the well-known and friendly environment that he or she spent years building.

A life at home, where the person's condition doesn't receive constant supervision, can, however, mean a life at risk. The intimate and familiar home surroundings are little consolation if some particular disability exists or if personal experience in self-care is lacking, as is the case with Harvey. A disability may have been caused by a physical affliction, an accident, the effects of aging, or even a drastic lack of experience in a certain area. Here we will concentrate on the last two examples as they related to an elder remaining at home unsupervised versus entering a permanent care program (e.g., a nursing home or assisted living arrangement).

The effects of aging are well publicized. Possible memory deficiency, loss of mobility, and absence of needed medical care are terms all too frequently used when describing the common traits of aging. Although an elder might not need constant supervision or care (e.g., in a nursing home or assisted living environment), the effects of aging can lead to a life at risk unless these effects can be countered by appropriate action. It is important for loved ones, care providers, and neighbors to be aware of potential problems and possible solutions in the event that an elder chooses to remain at home. Great care must be taken to reinforce and support this decision, while at the same time minimizing the risks the elder may encounter.

Taking care of all the bills, making sure that all health coverage is up to date and complete, and maintaining investments and savings is not always an easy task, even for those experienced in doing so. For a man or woman in Harvey's situation, these tasks may seem incomprehensible if not insurmountable. Unfortunately, there are thousands upon thousands of Harveys—or Harriets—in the United States.

I hope to assist in identifying problems, looking for potential solutions, and then choosing courses of action to overcome these problems. This chapter concludes with a list of national organizations that may be of assistance in the event that local resources are not available or helpful.

Information will be offered on:

- Medicare and senior health insurance,

- Social Security and other sources of income,

- problem solving and communicating,

- managing daily life, and

- finding organizations and individuals who can help.

Whether from the perspective of a family member, a concerned friend, or a caring neighbor, I hope to answer some of the major and most common questions that are raised when an elder chooses to remain living in the general community.

MEDICARE AND SENIOR HEALTH INSURANCE

Proper healthcare becomes more and more important with age. In an effort to ensure that all elders of the United States have access to medical care, the U.S. Congress passed the Medicare Bill of 1965. This law gives a form of medical insurance to all citizens when they reach age sixty-five. Although it does not provide 100 percent coverage, it does cover most of the costs associated with hospitalization and "necessary" outpatient treatment.

Medicare consists of two parts: part A (Hospitalization) and part B (Outpatient Care). Both have deductibles as well as limitations of coverage. To receive part B coverage (Supplemental Health Insurance), the elder must pay a monthly premium ($36.60 in 1988).[1] Figure 1 gives a brief breakdown of the definitions and limitations of Medicare coverage as of 1993.

Figure 1

MEDICARE COVERAGE 1993[2]

PART A: HOSPITALIZATION

- All "medically necessary" inpatient hospital care for up to 90 days during the benefit period. For the first 60 days part A pays for all covered services except the first $676. From the 60th to 90th day part A pays for all covered services except $169 per day.

- Up to 100 days a year in a skilled nursing facility (nursing home). For the first 20 days all covered services are paid. From day 21 to day 100 part A pays for all covered services except for $84.50 per day.

- Visits by nurses or other health workers (not doctors) from a home health agency for up to 21 consecutive days.

- Hospice care for terminally ill patients

PART B: SUPPLEMENTARY MEDICAL INSURANCE

- 80%–100% coverage for all "reasonable" charges (consult the care provider first, as this definition changes periodically), minus a once yearly deductible of $100

There is one major reason why it is important to understand exactly what Medicare will and will not cover. Most people find it necessary to supplement Medicare insurance with health insurance from a private company (often referred to as a carrier or underwriter). This insurance usually will not only prevent total financial devastation from a catastrophic medical situation (e.g., stroke, heart attack, organ transplant), but also it will provide stability in terms of financial planning (i.e., fixed bills without many variations or unexpected costs). Private insurance usually pays the Medicare deductibles and matches the partial Medicare payments, resulting in little or no out-of-pocket expense for the senior.

Private insurance may be expensive, however, and it usually gets more expensive with age. This expense, though, is basically set in stone and cannot increase unless it is a rate increase affecting all people in a specific category (for example, all people of the same sex, or all those of a particular age). These general rate increases are usually well-publicized, and preparations can be made far enough in advance of the anticipated increased expense to reduce the likelihood of major disruptions in the household budget. Catastrophic medical circumstances usually cannot be foreseen, though, and in some cases medical bills can approach half a million dollars. This huge amount, though Medicare may pay 80, 90, or even 98 percent of the bills, may be enough to seriously jeopardize the financial stability of even the most well-planned retirement unless Medicare is properly supplemented with private health insurance.

Surprising as it may seem, a local insurance agent may be the best resource for advice on financial planning. Special care must be taken, however, to ensure that the elder is either making a cautious, well-informed decision about his or her financial situation or that a concerned care provider is assisting with the process. Most insurance agencies offer free consultations, at which time they review the most recent Medicare and health-insurance laws (they change just about every year). Because of the frequent changes in Medicare, it is very difficult to offer exact advice on financial planning. The caregiver should make every effort to use the resources that are near or within the elder's community.

Another benefit to actually having a trustworthy insurance agent is that the "buck can be passed" to him or her insofar as processing insurance claims is concerned. Handling Medicare and other insurance claims is not very difficult; it is just important to do them in an orderly and timely fashion. Many insurance agencies provide a claims-processing service at little or no cost. Although the elder and his or her family may decide to take responsibility for filing all claims with Medicare and the private insurance company, allowing someone else to perform this duty—a professional whose job is insurance—can greatly reduce an often worrisome burden.

On the other hand, if total responsibility for maintaining all claims is taken by the elder and/or the caregiver (i.e., family member or friend), processing claims is rather easy. Usually it is only required that the medical bills be mailed to the insurance agency or to the Medicare processing center. Sometimes, the hospital or the specific clinic involved may perform this duty. In either case, prompt attention to all medical bills and insurance claims is important to ensure a quick resolution to any problems that may arise in the process (which, unfortunately, is not an uncommon occurrence).

In general, current knowledge of Medicare rules and coverages is tremendously important in choosing a health insurance supplement and in maintaining consistent, affordable healthcare coverage. This information is available at nearly any healthcare facility, government public service office, or insurance agency. Either the elder and the caregiver must be up to date on the continuing changes in the system, or the assistance of a trained professional must be enlisted. In choosing a professional agent, care must be taken to ensure trustworthiness and competence. (This person is responsible for the elder's well-being!) Shop around for the best agent and the best insurance rates without sacrificing coverage or service. If this is done properly and a responsible, caring agent is chosen, or if the changes in Medicare policy are continually monitored by the caregiver, the burden to the elder and to those offering assistance will be substantially lessened.

SOCIAL SECURITY AND OTHER SOURCES OF INCOME

The government has taken steps not only to provide for the health of elders, but also to guarantee some monthly income. The amount of the monthly Social Security check is determined by a formula that takes into consideration the maximum amounts of Social Security Tax (i.e., FICA tax) withheld from an individual's wages over the period when the individual was in the workforce. Currently, to receive maximum Social Security benefits, the individual must have paid a qualifying amount of Social Security taxes for a period of ten years while working. Partial benefits can be awarded in the event of early retirement (age sixty-two) or of disability. In the event of the death of a spouse, the larger of the husband's or wife's Social Security check should be received by the surviving spouse.

Although the monthly Social Security check to an individual may be relatively small (the average monthly benefit in December 1990 was $603),[3] it is the government's responsibility to make certain that the payment is sufficient to cover (or at least largely supplement) the cost of living. Therefore, these payments are raised periodically through what are called C.O.L.A.s—a Cost of Living Adjustments—which are tied to the general rise in consumer prices as reflected in the Consumer Price Index.

There are methods of knowing exactly how much an individual has paid into the government's Social Security fund and of determining if the correct benefits are being accrued. By contacting the U.S. Social Security Administration (U.S. Department of Health and Human Services), these inquiries can be made.*

In order to ensure a healthy and comfortable retirement, it is hoped that the individual has managed to save some money to add to the Social Security allowance. Unfortunately, this is not always the case. To compound the problem, Medicare does not cover the full costs of healthcare. For this reason it is necessary for the financial matters of an elder to be closely monitored, if not completely managed, by an informed and caring party.

Social Security may be supplemented with part-time employment, but after a certain amount has been earned, Social Security recipients are taxed. In 1990, for instance, $1 was deducted from the monthly benefit for every additional $3 earned above $9,720.[3] For this reason careful thought should be given to just how much part- or full-time work is actually necessary to supplement Social Security. A part-time job can be very rewarding, offering positive distractions from daily life, and it can serve as a constructive method of utilizing free time. Extra employment after retirement may not be required or desired, but at least it is a feasible means of increasing monthly income in some cases, and should be considered as such.

Other sources of income include retirement allowances (e.g., 401Ks, annuities, pensions) which may have been established during the person's, or his or her spouse's, years of employment. By the time the elder has retired, these allowances should be for the most part set in stone, although some extra withdrawals may be allowed (sometimes with penalty) in the event of personal hardship or emergency. If such action seems the only method of balancing monthly expenditures,

---

*The telephone number and address for this organization can be found in the Appendix at the end of this chapter.

thoughtful consultation and assistance should be sought from the officer or agent in charge of the specific account. The phone number or address at which to reach this individual should be located on any monthly statement or check stub received from the organization in charge of managing the account.

In searching for additional sources of income, do not forget potential family support, extra government assistance (e.g., food stamps, various personal assistance programs) or local charitable organizations. A phone call to the local chamber of commerce or church organization may be a good start in learning what the local community may have to offer in terms of public services.* No qualified elder should ever feel sheepish or self-conscious about making such inquiries. These are government and private agencies whose job it is to help those who need a little assistance now and again. It's not a handout—it's your right as a taxpayer and as a human being.

PROBLEM SOLVING AND COMMUNICATING

Knowing the problems that may potentially arise when an elder chooses to remain at home is actually half of the battle. This knowledge is easy to find: just read any number of books or government supplements. What's tough is identifying a problem as a problem and then choosing the proper solution in an informed manner.

There are various reasons for this being the toughest stage of handling a problem. First and foremost, an elder may be unlikely to broadcast personal concerns or difficulties, as this could (in his or her eyes) endanger the continued opportunity of remaining at home. Elders sometimes feel that to admit they need some assistance is conceding that they might be unfit to stay on their own. Nothing could be farther from the truth. Everyone needs help some time, whether it be with balancing a checkbook or with choosing the best insurance plan. Nonetheless, an elder may become justifiably paranoid. Keep in mind, therefore, that when working with the affairs of someone else, care should be taken not to infringe upon his or her independence.

The elder might well be willing to admit openly that he or she has a problem, if only the person had an inkling that a problem exists. As you'll recall, this was one of the main problems in Harvey's case.

---

*Some of the organizations listed in the Appendix may also be able to direct you to organizations able to assist you in your search.

Since his wife had handled virtually all the family affairs, Harvey was totally in the dark about what had been done, what was being done, and what should be done concerning his financial and other affairs. In cases like these, it is up to an observant party to identify telltale signs or clues that something may be amiss.

These clues may not always be openly broadcast: usually they are subtle, but descriptive disturbances or occurrences (figure 2). A mailbox brimming with mail, even though it is clear that the elder is home; frequent phone calls (when the observer is in the elder's home) which are short and where the elder answers quickly, in an irritated manner, or long phone calls that seem to confuse or distress the elder may all be signs that some personal matters are being neglected and unknown consequences are being faced. More obvious indicators of potential financial trouble are actual or threatened repossession of goods, or collection notices scattered in the mail. Since an elder may not always know exactly if a situation is serious or not (e.g., late bills, expiring insurance, etc.) and may not even admit it if he or she did know, a special effort should be made to observe the person's affairs closely, without violating the elder's private "space."

Figure 2

TELLTALE SIGNS THAT SOMETHING MAY BE WRONG

- Mailbox brimming with uncollected mail
- Collection notices in the mail
- Suspicious or threatening phone calls
- Threats of or actual repossession of property
- Frequent unrequested visitors
- Fraudulent solicitations (be on guard!)
- Utility (gas, electricity, water, or telephone) shutoff
- Empty cupboards/no grocery shopping

An example of a technique used to persuade an elder to allow help would be to approach the entire situation in an open and unintimidating manner, offering to help keep track of the bills, since you do the same for several other people—maybe a neighbor or aging parent or even your own family. This way it seems to the elder that you might enjoy helping out in such a manner, and since you apparently do it somewhat regularly, you're probably good at it.

There are some instances where an elder will openly accept such assistance, some situations where he or she will accept such an offer only after putting up a symbolic struggle, and some cases where an elder will not easily agree to receiving any help at all. The first two cases are relatively easy to deal with, given a little persistence, a positive approach, or even some "tough love." The last situation is trickier and requires some careful diplomacy and thoughtful action. Careful thought must be given to the decision to enter the private affairs of another person, even if the assistance is for his or her own good.*

MANAGING DAILY LIFE

Aside from just having to deal with major bills, many smaller but important details must be addressed. Food, clothing, and transportation must be figured into the monthly budget along with the larger items of health insurance, monthly rent or house payment, and any other fixed bills or payments. These necessities can be lumped into a monthly budget but require the same watchful eye. It makes no sense to economize on one of these items when another may be worsened. (For example, cutting back on food may save a few dollars but the potential health risks are too great.) By the same token, some of these expenses, unless closely monitored, can easily get out of hand.

For these reasons, a moderately supervised monthly budget is a good idea. A budget should be flexible enough to allow the elder some sense of independence, but strict enough to ensure that the elder is at little risk of making a mistake or miscalculation that could jeopardize his or her financial security. When possible, it might be a good idea to set up accounts with stores frequented by the older person. Transactions can be closely monitored each month and easier lump payments can be made.

---

*For further information on communicating and dealing with uncooperative people, consult chapter 1 in this volume.

An additional benefit to such financial arrangements is the familiarity that starts to build when a person regularly visits one establishment. Friendly smiles and conversations are exchanged; shopping, dining out, or relaxing can be done in familiar surroundings; and, equally important, the employees of the establishment (in the case of a smaller facility) may come to know the elder on a first-name basis and even provide some candid assistance or supervision. A store clerk might be able to alert someone in the event that danger signals or irregularities become evident in the elder's behavior. The ability to meet people, to make friends, and to be in well-known surroundings may very well be the biggest benefit to making credit/charge account arrangements.

Once the elder has consented to allow help in formulating a budget, various questions remain: What should be put in the budget? How much should be spent? What might have been forgotten? Figure 3 shows a list of items that may or may not be required on every budget, but should be carefully considered for all budgets. This list may help people as a guide to setting up their own lists for subsequent budgets.

Figure 3

BRAINSTORMING POSSIBLE BUDGET ITEMS

Household Items

- Rent or Mortgage Payments
- Home Owner's Insurance
- Parking Fees (if any)
- Groceries
- Household Supplies

- Utilities
- Home/Yard Maintenance (mowing, painting, snow removal, cleaning services)
- Home decorations/adornment

Personal Items

- Health Insurance
- Personal Supplies (hygiene products, *medications*!)

- Transportation (car, auto insurance, maintenance)
- Clothes

Miscellaneous Items

- Entertainment (dining out, movies, books, relaxation, recreation)

- Travel

- Seasonal Activities (summer, winter, holidays)

- Periodical subscriptions

- Gifts (grandchildren, family, friends, neighbors)

- Vacationing

- Charitable Support (religious or other contributions)

The list in figure 3 may not be complete, but it should help to demonstrate the wide variety of items potentially in a budget.

After a list of likely budget items has been made, thought should be given to exactly how much money can be spent each month. A good suggestion might be to start with a fixed amount in the budget account, $500 for instance, and/or to adhere to a spending cap of 90 percent to 95 percent of the after-tax monthly income. This is the equivalent of saving 5 percent to 10 percent per month. The amount saved can be viewed as a safety or a buffer against unforeseen problems or mistakes, or it may serve as a "fun" account that grows until an alternate activity (i.e., a trip, cruise, "frivolous" purchase) may be allowed. Figure 4 illustrates how to construct a budget.

Figure 4

A SAMPLE BUDGET

Monthly Social Security Check $500.00
Monthly Pension/Retirement Plan Check 400.00
Interest from Savings (per month)...........................100.00
Assistance from Family (per month)..........................100.00

TOTAL INCOME PER MONTH $1100.00

A spending cap of 90% per month leaves $990 to be spent each month, while $110 is saved.

$$\$1100 \times 0.90 = \$990$$
$$\$1100 - \$990 = \$110$$

A spending cap of 95% per month leaves $1045 to be spent each month, while $55 is saved.

$$\$1100 \times 0.95 = \$1045$$
$$\$1100 - \$1045 = \$55$$

This sample budget continues by demonstrating how to figure monthly expenditures (see figure 5).

Figure 5

SAMPLE BUDGET (CONT.)

Expenses

Money Available to Spend (Income minus
    mandatory savings from figure 4).....................$1045.00
Savings (5% of monthly income) 55.00
Rent/Housing 300.00
Utilities: Electricity 25.00
          Heat/Gas 25.00
          Telephone (w/o long distance) 20.00
          Water/sewer/sanitation.............................20.00
Groceries 80.00
Home/Yard Maintenance.....................................40.00
Household Supplies...20.00
Supplemental Health Insurance 85.00
Transportation (gas, car insurance, parking) 150.00
Personal Supplies (hygiene, medications) 100.00
Entertainment 30.00
Gifts (grandchildren, greeting cards, etc.) 50.00
Charitable contributions 25.00

Miscellaneous (subscriptions, "fun" money) 20.00

TOTAL MONTHLY EXPENDITURES $1045.00

Almost everyone has experience in making and executing some type of budget. The purpose of this sample budget is to suggest the diversity and nature of a typical budget for an elderly person. This sample budget may not be typical, but it illustrates some different sources of funding and, subsequently, a varied breakdown of expenditures. Most budgets may not have the same characteristics, but most elements of the sample budget will be part of any budget.

Certain budgetary items, however, cannot be neglected. For instance, grandparents love to spend money on their children and grandchildren and should be allowed to do so. In addition, money should be set aside to enable the elder to hire someone to perform difficult or inconvenient tasks, such as yard maintenance, snow removal, or even grocery delivery. In fact, a weekly arrangement could be made with the local grocery store allowing the elder to call in a list and have the items delivered. The elder actually gets the groceries he or she needs, and the billing is orderly and convenient.

ADVICE TO THE CAREGIVER

By this time the caregiver should have at least a basic understanding of the rudimentary financial aspects of home care for the elderly. With some guidance, those concerned for the welfare of elders should be able to handle a difficult situation themselves or make use of available resources. If local resources are insufficient to solve a particular problem, help can be found in the attached Appendix, "Finding Organizations and Individuals Who Can Help."

First, let's summarize advice to caregivers when dealing with an elder's financial matters. This can be outlined in simple, straightforward terms.

Figure 6

ADVICE TO THE CAREGIVER

- Be observant of potentially neglected matters on the part of the elder, including:

    (a) unopened or unanswered mail,

    (b) unpaid bills,

    (c) various insurance coverages lapsing,

    (d) claims to Medicare or insurance not being filed.

- Frequently attempt to ascertain the elder's awareness of current financial matters:

    (a) Occasionally discuss insurance, investments, etc.

    (b) Be conscious of an "I don't know"/"I don't care" attitude.

- Be careful to protect the elder's autonomy and personal privacy, but at the same time be ready to intervene after the various methods of communication have been exhausted:

    (a) Help the elder to formulate a budget.

    (b) Oversee income and expenditures, separating the necessary from the unnecessary.

    (c) Ensure that all potential income resources are being utilized, that Medicare and insurance paperwork is up to date, and that the appropriate Social Security payments are being received.

    (d) When necessary, have the elder's important mail and other accounts forwarded to your address and telephone.

APPLICATIONS TO SPECIFIC SITUATIONS

Case Study 1: Solving Harvey's Situation

Harvey's neighbors contacted his sons about their concerns regarding Harvey's health and general well-being. His sons, in turn, took part of their vacation time to come see their father for several days. In addition to spending some good family time together, the sons collected all of Harvey's mail, bills, investment documents, insurance information, and Medicare paperwork. After discovering through gentle conversation that Harvey was for the most part unaware of his financial situation, his sons asked him if he would let them manage his finances.

Naturally, Harvey hit the roof at first, believing that these actions might be the first steps toward moving him into a home for the aged. His sons reassured him time and time again, however, that by taking care of his finances, they would be making certain that he would be able to live on his own. With further assurance they also convinced him that he was no burden on them, that making sure their *only* father was secure was their only concern. Harvey then agreed (happily on the inside, because what they said actually made sense after he put his pride aside).

Harvey agreed to have his regular bills and important account information forwarded to his eldest son's home, since Harvey was pretty tired of seeing it pile up ominously on the old table next to the phone in the living room. His sons then "reintroduced" their father to his neighbors and found out that an elderly gentleman three doors down also recently lost his wife. He and this new acquaintance got along rather well, and arrangements were made for mutual grocery shopping excursions and entertainment. A comfortable budget was formulated, since Harvey's investments and retirement account was still intact and, luckily, no insurance coverage had lapsed. A trip to the local physician, spurred along by his sons, proved beneficial, as Harvey's medication was changed; soon his forgetfulness decreased and his activity level increased, so much so that his sons were able to teach him the simple procedure of sending in medical claims to his insurance company.

All of the bases had been touched: Harvey's bills and regular notices were being taken care of; all coverages were up to date and being maintained; Harvey's basic need swere well tended to; and, to top it off, Harvey began entering the outside world again, free to enjoy his retirement a little more.

Not all cases will work out as well as Harvey's. Some situations

will be much more difficult to manage, with fewer resources and les
assistance from family members.

Case Study: Squeaking by on a Tight Budget

Pat lost her husband, Frank, five years ago. He had been a proud man, insisting on handling all of the finances as well as earning all of the money. They had been comfortable, enjoying a pleasant home on a beautiful lake, as they approached retirement. Gradually, however, the situation became worse.

Frank had slowly become more forgetful, losing track of some payments and generally mismanaging money as he worked less and less upon entering retirement. By the time they actually retired, the couple was bankrupt: Frank had been unable to make enough money to pay the bills while not yet receiving Social Security. The bankruptcy wiped out all investments and savings, as well as a good portion of their possessions. They moved from the lake to an apartment in a small town nearby.

Frank died a few years later from many complications which Pat knew to be mainly attributed to the distress he felt at not being able to deal with his money problems and not turning to anyone for help. When he was gone, Pat literally had nothing except one monthly Social Security check.

Pat enjoyed keeping busy and worked part-time in a local specialty shop. The money she earned was enough to pay some monthly bills and buy food and occasional odds and ends. In general, however, money was tight. Her own health was gradually failing, and caring friends began hinting that she might benefit from entering an assisted living facility. With no living relatives, Pat had the concern of these friends, whom she respected, but she feared such places and refused to consider the possibility. The medical bills kept piling up due to an inexpensive insurance plan that did not cover all the expenses, and a large monthly rent payment stared her in the face. Pat was gradually sliding into more money problems.

A neighbor and close friend, Mildred, saw what was happening and decided to help. She shopped around for a Medicare supplement for Pat that would give her full coverage, even if it cost her a little bit more. She met a terrific agent named John, who later met with Pat and in clear, uncomplicated terms explained to both of them the benefits of a different policy. Pat switched, as she had no serious preexisting medical conditions. The new policy was more expensive, but she actually ended up saving a sizable sum of money now that her new policy would cover most of the 20 percent Part B copayment.

Pat then had her monthly rent reduced somewhat by agreeing with her landlord to perform some light maintenance to the building (sweeping sidewalks, dusting rails) in an effort to keep busy. With these two savings, Pat could more easily afford her expenses and even had some money left over each month. The insurance agent, processed all of Pat's claims and was even able to provide some other financial management advice.

With the help of Mildred and John, Pat was able to continue living on her own, while keeping a strong sense of independence. Without their assistance, Pat probably would have gone down the same path as her husband. In many such cases elders will have most of their faculties in place; they simply need a little caring guidance and support. The last thing they need or want is to be dependent on someone else.

Needless to say, one should only spend as much money each month as one receives, but this may not always be possible. Too many horror stories are told about the concessions people must make when there is not enough money to meet their basic needs. Since every case is somewhat different, the best solution to individual problems lies in the available resources: local government agencies, associations of retired persons, friends who have overcome similar problems, and the like.

The appendix gives a brief list of national organizations involved with some aspect of the aging population. These organizations may be able to give some direct assistance or describe the availability of any local or regional resources.

APPENDIX

Finding Organizations or Individuals Who Can Help

National Organizations:

- The American Association of Retired Persons (AARP)
  1909 K. Street NW
  Washington, D.C. 20049
  (202) 872-4700

- National Clearinghouse on Aging
  330 Independence Avenue S.W.
  Washington, D.C. 20201
  (202) 245-2158

- National Institute on Aging
  Federal Building, Room 6C12
  9000 Rockville Pke
  Bethesda, MD 20892
  (301) 496-1752

- Social Security Administration
  6401 Security Boulevard
  Baltimore, MD 21235
  (301) 594-1234

- National Clearinghouse for Family Planning
  PO Box 2225
  Rockville, MD 20852
  (301) 881-9400

Local Organizations (check your yellow or white pages)

- State Department of Health and Human Service

- County Office of Human Services or Social Services

- A local senior center.

NOTES

1. Social Security Administration, U.S. Department of Health and Human Services (consumer information publication), 1993.
2. U.S. Department of Health and Human Services (consumer informational bulletin), 1993.
3. *The World Almanac and Book of Facts: 1992.* New York: Pharos Books, 1991. Mark S. Hoffman (ed.), pp. 689–90.

ADDITIONAL REFERENCES

Kelly-Hayes, Margaret; Allen M. Jette; Philip A. Wolf; Ralph B. D'Agostino; and Patricia M. Odell. "Functional Limitation and Disability among Elders in the Framingham Study," *The American Journal of Public Health* (June 1992): 841–45.
Larue, Gerald, and Rich Bayly. *Long-Term Care in an Aging Society.* Buffalo, N.Y.: Prometheus Books, 1992, pp. 93–117.

4

The Importance of Nutrition at Home

Elizabeth A. Wegner

Proper nutrition is one of the most important criteria for an elder adult to remain healthy. People with good eating habits will feel healthy and more alert, and have more energy. Meals should be balanced and contain food from the basic food groups: meats, dairy products, fruits and vegetables, breads and cereals, and fats and oils.

A balanced diet cannot always be obtained if an elder has a mental or physical handicap and is living alone. Problems that could reduce food intake include paralysis (e.g., which occurs in stroke patients or arthritis sufferers), dementia (which occurs in persons with Alzheimer's disease), crippling (e.g., persons with arthritis), lack of coordination (e.g., persons with Parkinson's disease), and blindness (especially if the vision loss happened later in life).[1] These elders may not be able to shop for groceries or cook for themselves. Some may forget to eat, or may not eat, because they are "just not very hungry." Vitamin and mineral deficiencies may result, and the body's ability to fight disease could be seriously compromised. Under such conditions, an aged body may not be able to recover as quickly—or not as all—when it encounters a disease.

A possible solution to this nutrition problem could be the preparation of meals by a caregiver. The caregiver must create meals that are pleasing to the palate while avoiding empty calories from foods high in fat and low in nutritional value.

Older adults may require a change in nutritional habits, which arises as a result of the extent of the aging process, the physical and chemical environments, activity levels, existing health problems, current medications, and alcohol intake.[2] The 1989 Surgeon General's Report stressed that changes in physiology, psychology, economic situation, and social circumstances that occur as we age can have an effect on the body's need for certain nutrients.

Currently, it is not conclusively known if older adults need to increase or decrease their nutrient intake. It is known that if older people maintain their physical activity, either by regular exercise or performing physical work, their food-energy requirements are related to their energy expenditure, not unlike younger individuals.[3] The total energy production per square meter of body surface falls with advancing age. The decrease may be due to the loss of metabolizing tissue or to the loss of physical activity.[4]

Age-related changes in body composition as well as reduction in cardiac, respiratory, hepatic, and renal function may influence nutritional needs.[5] To maintain nutrient intakes high enough for good health, older adults will need to consume diets of higher nutrient-to-energy ratios.[6]

Listed below are protein, vitamin, and mineral requirements, recommended for older adults to maintain a health. Caregivers to older adults should consult this list to become familiar with what foods contain specific nutrients, the problems if a diet is deficient in a certain area, the special needs of elders, and the Recommended Dietary Allowances per day.

PROTEIN REQUIREMENTS

Protein is available in many foods and should be included in the diet one to two times per day. Protein can be found in milk, cheese, chicken, beef, pork, fish, and peas. Protein deficiency can occur in people who are on a starvation regimen while undergoing the stress of infection, injury, or surgery.[7] Also, a deficiency can develop if a disease prevents the ingestion of protein or if an individual is extensively burned.

Specific protein requirements for older adults cannot be recommended, because there is not enough information available on this population. The current protein requirement for the average adult is 0.8 milligrams per kilogram of body weight.[8]

VITAMIN REQUIREMENTS

Vitamin A

Vitamin A is required for normal skin tissues and to maintain vision.[9] This vitamin has been identified as a protective agent against cancer, and it helps to resist the formation of tumors.[10] Carotenoids are vitamin A precursors found in yellow and dark-green vegetables. Beta-carotene has been found to have the highest provitamin activity. The conversion of carotenoids to retinol (plasma vitamin A) is performed in the mucous membranes of the intestines. Carotenoids are also able to enhance cellular immune responses, inhibit the growth of metated cells, reduce the extent of DNA damage, and have provided protection against light-induced skin cancer in experimental animals.[11] Vitamin A that is preformed is found in dairy products, including milk, cheese, butter, and ice cream.[12] Rich food sources of the vitamin include liver, eggs, and fish (such as herrings, sardines, and tuna).[13]

There is no general agreement as to whether aging affects plasma retinol values.[14] In view of the increasing evidence of a need for carotenoids to lessen cancer risk, it is recommended that the intake of vegetable sources of these forms of vitamin A be maintained at an adequate level.[15] The Recommended Dietary Allowance (RDA) of vitamin A is 1,000 micrograms per day for men and 800 for women.

Vitamin D

Vitamin D, in its metabolically active form, is required for calcium absorption and for calcium release from bones so that calcium levels in the blood are maintained within normal limits.[16] Vitamin D is formed through a series of reactions after the skin is exposed to sunlight.[17] There is evidence that older adults may need additional vitamin D due to the bone loss that occurs with aging. The RDA of vitamin D for both men and women is 5 micrograms of cholecalciferol (a precursor to vitamin D) or 200 IU of vitamin D.

Vitamin K

Vitamin K is required for the synthesis of blood clotting factors and is required for normal blood coagulation.[18] A deficiency of vitamin K can lead to hemorrhaging into the skin, called purpura.[19] Foods rich in vitamin K include leafy green vegetables such as spinach, broccoli, and brussels sprouts.[20]

There is little evidence that older adults need more vitamin K than younger adults if they are eating the proper foods. If elders are ingesting antibiotics or mineral oils over a long period of time, synthesis and absorption of vitamin K can be affected.[21] The RDA of vitamin K is 1 microgram per day.

Vitamin E

Vitamin E has been proposed as an anti-oxidant that can slow down or prevent the aging process.[22] Reactive forms of oxygen have been implicated in certain disease processes prevalent in older adults such as chronic inflammatory diseases, radiation damage, and cancer. The reactive oxygen forms are generated by exposure to light and/or chemicals in the environment or in the diet.[23] Therefore, anti-oxidant vitamins can protect older adults against disease due to carcinogenic environmental agents.[24] Some anti-oxidant vitamins are E, C, and carotenoids.

Vitamin E can be found in vegetable oils, grains, seeds, and nuts. Vitamin E deficiency is rare in older adults and there is no definite evidence to suggest that the body's requirements for the vitamin increase as one ages.[25] The RDA of vitamin E is 10 milligrams alpha-tocopherol (wheat germ oil) equivalents for men and 8 for women. An alpha-tocopherol is one of four isomers of vitamin E.

Thiamin

Thiamin is required as a coenzyme in reactions needed for the intermediate metabolism of cells.[26] Natural food sources containing thiamin are cereal and cereal brans. In the United States, many baked goods and breakfast cereals are fortified with thiamin. The absorption of thiamin may be reduced with excessive alcohol or tea consumption.[27]

Thiamin levels of most healthy, independent older adults in the United States are adequate, but of those elders in long-term care facilities whose food intake is low, thiamin levels were also found to be low. The abuse of alcohol is a risk factor for thiamin deficiency.[28] The RDA of thiamin for people over age fifty-one is 1.2 milligrams per day.

Riboflavin

Riboflavin is required for oxidation-reduction reactions in its active coenzyme forms, flavin mononucleotide (FMW) and flavin dinucleotide (FAD).[29] Flavins are required for the metabolizing of drugs and for efficient energy use.[30] Riboflavin can be found in milk, cheese, yogurt, liver, and many breads and breakfast cereals.

Older adults may have riboflavin deficiency if their caloric intake is less than the recommended daily amount of 2,000 kilocalories of food energy. The RDA of riboflavin is 0.6 milligram per 1,000 kilocalories per day for men and women of all age groups.[31]

Niacin

Niacin can be found in chicken, peas, enriched whole wheat bread, fortified cereals, enriched rice, and bran muffins. The amount of niacin an older adult consumes varies with income: those who have more money generally are able to consume more animal protein.[32] There is no scientific basis for increasing the RDA of niacin for older adults.[33] The RDA of niacin is 15 milligrams for men, and 13 for women.

Folic Acid

Folic acid or folate can be found in fortified breakfast cereals and dark green, leafy vegetables. There have been some studies of institutionalized elders and those living on their own that have shown a high incidence of mild folate deficiency.[34] Signs of folate deficiency include a specific type of anemia and an organic brain syndrome characterized by mental confusion and loss of memory.[35]

Folate levels can be maintained if older adults consume the foods mentioned above. Currently, there is no recommendation to change the RDA of folate for older adults, now set an 200 micrograms for men and 180 for women.

Vitamin B$_6$

Vitamin B$_6$ can be found in many fortified cereals. A deficiency of this vitamin can be caused by drugs that neutralize its presence in the body. A few examples are isoniaazad (isonicotinic acid hydrazide, INH), cycloserine, L-dopa, or penecillamine.[36] Also, alcohol abuse can lead to a deficiency of vitamin B$_6$.[37]

There is some evidence that vitamin B$_6$ requirements increase with age.[38] There is presently not enough information to suggest that the RDA should be changed for older adults. The RDA of vitamin B$_6$ is 2.0 milligrams for men and 1.6 milligrams for women.

Vitamin C

Vitamin C can be found in citrus fruits, green vegetables, tomatoes, potatoes, and fortified cereals. A deficiency of this vitamin may lead to scurvy, which may include bleeding from the gums, delayed wound healing, and purpura.[39] Fatigue may also be related to lowered·vitamin C intake. High doses of aspirin may cause vitamin C depletion.[40]

There is currently no evidence of a change in absorption or metabolization of vitamin C with age, or any recommendation to change the RDA of vitamin C for older adults.[41] The RDA for vitamin C is 60 milligrams for both men and women.

MINERAL AND TRACE ELEMENT REQUIREMENTS

Calcium

Calcium is a very important mineral for older adults to consume because it is crucial to the development and maintenance of bone. Calcium-rich foods include milk, cheese, ice cream, and other dairy products.

Older adults need to consume more calcium than younger people, due to the following factors mentioned by Roe (1992). Age-related bone loss can be reduced by taking in more calcium. Severe bone loss is the underlying cause of fractures, which lead to disability and high health-care costs. Also, calcium absorption decreases with age, particularly in women after menopause. If an older adult becomes less active, bone loss may increase, calling for an increase in calcium consumption. The risk of hypertension may be decreased by increasing calcium intake.[42] The RDA of calcium is 800 milligrams per day. If a calcium supplement is taken, it should not be administered at mealtime; to do so could reduce the absorption of dietary folate and iron from foods eaten during the meal.[43] Too much calcium, on the other hand, can cause impaired kidney function, if taken in the form of calcium carbonate.

Iron

Iron is an important mineral in our diet and can be found in spinach, chicken, fish, and other animal proteins. Studies conducted on older persons living independent lives show a low frequency of iron deficiency anemia.[44] This may be due to the fact that the body's ability to store iron increases with age, and many older adults tend to consume more than 10 milligrams a day, which is the current RDA.[45] Iron deficiency anemia presents itself with the person feeling weak, pale, and out of breath. Low iron levels in the body can also be the result of severe bleeding caused by a peptic ulcer, bowel cancer, and chronic aspirin use.[46]

Zinc

Zinc is an important mineral for maintaining the immune system and for promoting the healing of wounds. Peas contain zinc, along with other needed nutrients. Be aware, however, that the absorption of zinc can be reduced if an older adult is consuming a recommended high-fiber diet.[47] Zinc deficiency can also occur if diets low in the mineral are consumed. There is still a need to reassess special dietary zinc guidelines for older adults.[48] The RDA for zinc is 15 milligrams a day.

CASE STUDIES

Mrs. Jenson, a ninety-year-old woman living independently, is not as mobile as she used to be, and now needs a walker to move about the house. Aside from her reduced mobility, Mrs. Jenson's appetite has not decreased in the least bit. She is used to having a large meal at noon, but is no longer able to prepare it herself.

For Mrs. Jenson, a caregiver could be hired to come into her house for a few hours at mealtime every day. The caregiver could purchase groceries or look into the availability of food shopping assistance in the area. The local Area Agency on Aging can be of great help in locating such a program. Groceries selected by Mrs. Jenson would allow healthy and filling meals to be prepared composed of her favorite dishes.

When food shopping assistance is utilized, the older adult may qualify for food stamps. The caregiver, a relative, or even a close friend in the neighborhood could contact the local Department of Social Services to take advantage of this right for the older adult.

When caring for older adults, special attention should be given to providing the proper amount of food from the four basic food groups: two servings of dairy products, one to two servings from the meat group, four servings of vegetables and fruits (which may include fruit juices), and four servings of cereals should be prepared each day.[49]

Those who assist the elderly should pay special attention to the elder's personal cleanliness and must not have any communicable diseases. If a caregiver, friend, or relative were to bring a virus or bacteria into the older adult's home, the elder may have a difficult time recovering from the illness. A conscious effort must be made to keep the working conditions sanitary.

*   *   *

Mrs. Smith lives in an assisted living apartment complex, a building where hired staff is available if needed. She chose not to be included in the meal program in the dining room, because she never feels hungry. Mrs. Smith does not feel the need to pay money for food she will not eat or may not even like.

The pleasure of eating may not be as great for an older adult. The person may not feel hungry, or the sense of taste may not be as acute. Variety is a key to preparing an elder person's meals. There are many ethnic and foreign foods that can be pleasing with extra spice for added flavor.

Mr. Johnson currently has his meals prepared by a caregiver through the hospital. He has experienced congestive heart failure and has always been overweight. Mr. Johnson needs to lower his sodium and cholesterol intake. Special care should be taken by the caregiver to see that his special requirements are met.

Mrs. Howel, a frail lady of eighty-three, lives alone in an apartment complex. She receives home healthcare through a fellow church member. Mrs. Howel has shown a marked weight loss the last several times she has been visited by her doctor. The physician recommended a high-calorie, low-fat diet to the caregiver.

Individuality is an important factor, because each elder is very different. For example, some need to lose weight, while others need to gain a few pounds or maintain their current weight. Also, some older adults need more or less of a certain vitamin or mineral due to their activity level or a disease process encountered. An individual diet should be planned by the caregiver for each special case. If possible, a dietitian should be consulted to coordinate meal plans for caregivers who work through an agency, or independently.

Common ailments and prescribed special diets, as listed by Daphne A. Roe in *Geriatric Nutrition,* are as follows:

1. Congestive heart failure—low-sodium diet

2. Atherosclerotic heart disease [hardening of the arteries]—low-cholesterol diet

3. Hypertension [high blood pressure]—low-sodium diet

4. Obesity—low-calorie diet

5. Diabetes—low-calorie, low-sugar diet

6. Renal failure [kidney failure]—low-protein diet

7. Cirrhosis [liver disease]—low-protein, low-sodium diet

8. Diverticulosis and diverticulitis [lesions in the colon]—low-fat diet

9. Constipation—high-fiber diet

10. Hiatus hernia—low-bulk diet

11. Cholecystitis [inflammation of the gall bladder] and chole-lithiasis [solid masses in the gall bladder]—low-fat, low cholesterol diet

12. Colostomy [artificial opening to void the colon]—low-fiber diet.[50]

Mrs. Peterson, an independently living seventy-year-old, was recently diagnosed with bone cancer. Moving about her house has become difficult due to the back brace she must wear. Preparing meals has become impossible, because of the pain she experiences while standing or walking. She has no relatives living nearby. Mr. Warner suffers from severe arthritis (the wearing away of cartilage between bones at the joints) causing him serious pain when he moves about. He doesn't have enough money to hire a caregiver to come into his home and prepare his meals. Mr. Warner's grown children provide groceries for him, but lack the time to prepare any meals.

Many adult children of elder parents do not have the time needed to prepare healthy meals for their parents and often cannot afford to have someone come in and cook for their family member. A great social program called "Meals on Wheels" is available in nearly every community. This is a program that delivers nutritious meals to people who are unable to prepare food themselves. The meals have one-third the daily nutrients and calories needed for an adult. Individuals qualify to receive the meals if they are homebound; sixty-five years of age or older; or a low-income, younger handicapped person. In an effort to keep the cost of meals low, volunteers deliver them to elders. Donations or a minimal cost per meal is requested, but this varies with the income level of the person receiving the service. Packaged meals are also delivered for those days when the deliverer can't make it to the destination. These meals can be heated in the oven for a specific period of time and then eaten. Recipients of the meals may cancel their delivery if they will not be home, thus no food is wasted.

Miss Jorgensen has lived alone all her life. Recently, her vision has deteriorated due to cataracts. She cannot see well enough to prepare her own meals, so her neighbor has volunteered to cook for her. Miss Jorgenson's neighbor, as kind as she is, lacks the education necessary to prepare meals that contain the recommended dietary allowances. Nutrition education programs are available for older adults, caregivers, or the children of an older adult to gain the knowledge necessary to prepare healthy and delicious meals. The programs are designed to give dietary knowledge and counseling. Special diets can be personally designed for the special care of particular older adults. Such nutrition education programs may be provided at congregate meal sites, senior centers, in churches, in domiciliary care facilities, and in long-term care facilities.[51]

Mrs. Kallahan, a recent widow, is a seventy-five-year-old woman who is very lonely. Having a bus stop across the street from her apartment building, she has access to any part of the city. Since her husband died, Mrs. Kallahan often wishes she could have people over to dine with her.

One solution to this problem could be dining at a congregate meal facility, a location where many senior citizens go to enjoy a hot and nutritious meal. Under the 1973 Amendment of Title VII of the Older Americans Act of 1965, the Nutrition Program for Older Americans was established. This program, funded by the government, provides a national food program for older adults.[52] Funds were made available to each of the fifty states and some American territories. Each state is responsible for locating older adults who may need the services and appropriating funds to the meal sites. Now, Title III of the Older Americans Act is responsible for the meals in each community. The meal sites may be located at senior centers, religious establishments, schools, public housing, restaurants, or community centers.[53] Title III requires that at least one hot meal is served per day and that one-third of the recommended dietary allowances be provided in that meal. Also, the meal sites must be located in areas easily accessible to many older adults. The congregate meal setting would not only offer balanced meals, but company for older adults at mealtime and the fulfillment of the need for socialization.

Dietary guidelines for the general population, including older adults, are listed below. These guidelines are transcribed from Daphne Roe's *Geriatric Nutrition* (1992) and are also stated in the National Research Council's monograph *Diet and Health* (1989). These guidelines should be followed by those who care for an older adult.

1. Reduce total fat intake to 30 percent or less of total calories.

2. Every day eat five or more servings of a combination of vegetables and fruits, especially green and yellow vegetables and citrus fruits.

3. Increase intake of complex carbohydrates to 55 percent of total calories. Include cereals which provide good sources of dietary fiber.

4. Maintain a moderate protein intake.

5. Balance food intake and physical activity to maintain appropriate body weight.

6. Do not consume alcohol.

7. Limit total daily intake of salt.

8. Maintain adequate calcium intake.

9. Avoid taking dietary supplements in excess of the RDA during any one day.

Eating can be pleasurable late in life, even if elders cannot prepare the food themselves. If a caregiver takes the time and effort to prepare tasty and healthy meals, the older adult will feel better and quite possibly look better. The Meals on Wheels program is available for older adults who do not have someone to cook for them. Variety, individuality, and a little bit of creativity can improve mealtime for any elder citizen.

NOTES

1. D. A. Roe, *Geriatric Nutrition,* 3d ed. (Englewood Cliffs, N.J.: Prentice Hall, Inc., 1992).
2. Ibid.
3. Ibid.
4. Exton-Smith 1972
5. Roe, *Geriatric Nutrition.*
6. Ibid.

7. C. E. Butterworth, Jr., and R. L. Weinsier, "Malnutrition in Hospitalized Patients: Assessment and Treatment," in *Modern Nutrition in Health and Disease,* 6th ed., edited by R. S. Goodhart and M. E. Shils (Philadelphia: Lee and Febiger, 1980), pp. 667–80.

8. Munro 1980

9. M. C. Linder, "Nutrition and Metabolism of Vitamins," in *Nutritional Biochemistry and Metabolism,* edited by M. C. Linder (New York: Elsevier North-Holland, Inc., 1985), pp. 102–110.

10. Y. H. Yupsa, "Retinoids and Tumor Promotion," in *Diet, Nutrition and Cancer: From Basic Research to Policy Implications* (New York: Alan R. Liss Publishers, Inc., 1983), pp. 95–109.

11. A. Benich and J. A. Olsen, "Biological Actions of Carotenoids," *FASEBJ* 3 (1989): 1972–32.

12. Roe, *Geriatric Nutrition.*

13. Watt and Merrill 1963

14. J. E. Kirk and W. Chieffi, "Vitamin Studies in Middle Aged and Old Individuals: I. The Vitamin A, Total Carotene, and Alpha and Beta Carotene Concentration in Plasma," *Journal of Nutrition* 36 (1948): 315–22; H. A. Rafsky, B. Newman, and N. Jollife, "A Study of the Carotene and Vitamin A Levels in the Aged," *Gastroenterology* 8 (1984): 612–15; H. A. Gillum, A. F. Morgan, and F. L. Sailer, "Nutritional Status of the Aging," *Journal of Nutrition* 55 (1955): 655–70.

15. Roe, *Geriatric Nutrition.*

16. Ibid.

17. Ibid.

18. J. W. Suitte and R. E. Olsen, "Vitamin K," in *Present Knowledge in Nutrition,* 5th ed. (Washington, D.C.: The Nutrition Foundation, 1984), pp. 241–59.

19. Roe, *Geriatric Nutrition.*

20. Suitte and Olsen, "Vitamin K."

21. Roe, *Geriatric Nutrition.*

22. Ibid.

23. Ibid.

24. Ibid.

25. Ibid.

26. Ibid.

27. V. Tanphaichitr and B. Wood, "Thiamin," in *Present Knowledge in Nutrition.*

28. F. L. Iber, J. P. Blass, M. Brin, and C. M. Leevy, "Thiamin in the Elderly: Relation to Alcoholism and to Neurological Degenerative Disease," *American Journal of Clinical Nutrition* 6 (1982): 1067–82.

29. Roe, *Geriatric Nutrition.*

30. Ibid.

31. Ibid.

32. Ibid.

33. P. J. Garry, J. S. Goodwin, W. C. Hunt, E. M. Hooper, and A. G. Leonard, "Nutritional Status in a Healthy Elderly Population: Dietary and Supplemental Intakes," *American Journal of Clinical Nutrition* 36 (1982): 319–31.

34. Roe, *Geriatric Nutrition.*

35. Ibid.

36. Ibid.

37. Lumeng and Li 1974

38. Garry et al., "Nutritional Status in a Healthy Elderly Population: Dietary and Supplemental Intakes"; and J. C. Guilland, B. Bereksi-Reguig, Lequeu, D. Moreau, J. Klepping, and D. Richard, "Evaluation of Pyridoxine Status among Aged Institutionalized People," *Journal of Vitamin and Nutritional Research* 54 (1984): 185–93.

39. Roe, *Geriatric Nutrition.*

40. G. Coffey and C. W. M. Wilson, "Ascorbic Acid Deficiency and Aspirin-Induced Haematemesis," *British Medical Journal* (1975): 208.

41. J. E. Kirk and W. Chieffi, "Vitamin Studies in Middle Aged and Old Individuals: XII. Hypovitaminemia C," *Journal of Gerontology* 8 (1953): 305–311.

42. D. A. McCarron, "Is Calcium More Important than Sodium in the Pathogenesis of Essential Hypertension?" *Hypertension* 7 (1985): 657–67.

43. Roe, *Geriatric Nutrition.*

44. P. R. Dallman, R. Yip, and C. Johnson, "Prevalance and Causes of Anemia in the United States, 1976–1980," *American Journal of Clinical Nutrition* 39 (1984): 437.

45. Cook, Finch, and Smith 1976 and Lynch et al.

46. Roe, *Geriatric Nutrition.*

47. Ibid.

48. Ibid.

49. Ibid.

50. Ibid.

51. Ibid.

52. Ibid.

53. Ibid.

ADDITIONAL REFERENCES

Bowman, B. B., and I. H. Rosenberg. "Assessment of the Nutritional Status of the Elderly," *American Journal of Clinical Nutrition* 35 (1982): 1142–51.

Newton, H. M. V., M. Sheltway, A. W. M. Hay, and B. Morgan, "The Relation Between Vitamin D_2 and D_3 in the Diet and Plasma $25(OH)D_2$ and $25(OH)D_3$ in Elderly Women in Great Britain," *American Journal of Clinical Nutrition* 41 (1985): 760–64.

5

Coping with Vision Loss

Elizabeth A. Wegner

Deteriorating vision is very likely in aging individuals. It is estimated that ten million adult Americans have lost their sight to some degree and that 43 percent of this number are age sixty-five or over.[1]

Good vision is important to maintaining an independent lifestyle. Basic tasks in the home are difficult for an elder with poor vision or one who has gone blind. A new relationship with space and time must be established. Vision loss challenges the ordering of perceptual categories and raises the question of personal competence.[2] Many changes in the eye that occur with age may pose a risk to an older individual living alone.

One change that occurs is flattening of the cornea, the most anterior portion of the eye. The cornea is the part of the eye that covers the pupil. This flattening leads to two points of focus instead of one, causing blurred vision.

A diagram of the eye is provided on page 81 to aid in understanding the anatomy of the eye and the disorders to which it is susceptible.

The iris, the part of the eye that controls the amount of light that falls on the retina by expanding or shrinking the pupil, may become rigid in older individuals.[3] This rigidity causes a smaller pupil, resulting in the need for more light that many elders request. The cause of this problem is not yet known.

The lens of the eye may lose some flexibility of thickness and curvature, resulting in *presbyopia,* commonly referred to as "aging eyes." It is the most common eye change as people grow older, usually having its onset after the age of forty.[4] This condition inhibits the eye's capacity

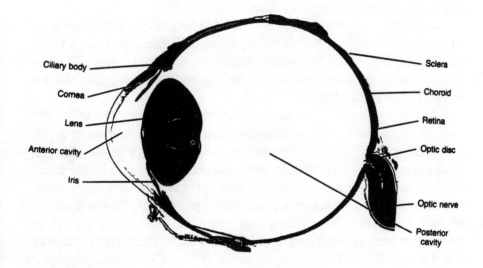

to focus on near objects, causing the common need for bifocals.[5] Symptoms of presbyopia are blurred vision at a normal reading distance, burning of the eye, and possibly a gritty feeling.[6]

Many elders develop *cataracts,* a whitish haze in the lens of the eye. A cataract sufferer sees images as if looking through dirty glasses. It is estimated that 95 percent of adults over the age of sixty-five have cataracts to some degree.[7] A person with cataracts needs more light passing through the smaller pupil, but light that is not too bright. Cataracts can be removed through surgery: the faulty lens is removed and replaced by the implantation of an intraocular lens. Great improvement of vision is sited in most cases.

Cataracts may be able to be prevented through diet: the consumption of foods rich in vitamin C is recommended. Examples of such foods are citrus fruits, green vegetables, tomatoes, and cantaloupe. The risk of developing cataracts increases with cigarette smoking and the exposure to ultraviolet light.[8]

Another change that occurs is that the *sclera* (the "white" of the eye) becomes less elastic, accumulates fatty deposits, and turns a yellowish color, which disturbs circulation and can cause *glaucoma* (internal ocular pressure). "Glaucoma is a progressive disease caused by too much pressure within the eye that blinds more people than any other single eye disease."[9] Glaucoma is caused by "faulty plumbing": the eye produces its own liquid rich in nutrients and when the eye cannot get rid of this as fast as is is produced, a buildup occurs.[10] The internal pressure can damage the retina and optic nerve fibers. Over time, peripheral vision decreases and night vision can be impaired.[11] Vision loss to glaucoma cannot be regenerated, but currently there is a technique for early detection of this pressure buildup.

Stanford University ophthalmologist Dr. Louis Roloff and photographer Jim Taskett have developed a technique to detect glaucoma up to two years earlier than previous methods.[12] "By photographing the optic nerve fibers—1,000,000 hair-like strands lining the back of the eye that are responsible for vision—as little as a 10 percent loss of fibers may be able to be detected."[13] This new technique enables doctors to stop the disease before the patient's vision is impaired. If detected early, glaucoma can be controlled with new medication in the form of eyedrops.

A disease called *macular degeneration* is the leading cause of blindness among older adults.[14] Macular degeneration is a destruction of the *macula lutea,* a tiny area at the center of the retina where day vision is the most distinct.[15] The retina loses resolving power, the ability to see fine details, along with the ability to adapt to the dark.

Signs of macular degeneration include blurred central vision, distortions of straight lines, and double vision.[16] Macular degeneration can be caused by exposure to ultraviolet light for a long period of time. Older adults should be careful to wear a good pair of sunglasses when exposed to sunlight. In addition, a diet containing zinc and vitamin E may help to protect the macula and retina, respectively.[17] Early detection of this problem is important, and, in some cases, treatment can be effective.

Older adults may experience something called *dry eyes.* The term is self-explanatory: the eyes fail to produce enough tears and may become scratchy and dry. Dry eyes in women can be caused by the change in estrogen levels that occur with aging; all elders with this condition may find that its presence is the result of the use of certain medications, or possibly due to arthritis.[18] Artificial tears purchased from a drug store can help to relieve the scratchy feeling, but these tears should not be confused with over-the-counter eyedrops that relieve red and tired eyes; the latter products are vasoconstrictors (which narrow the blood vessels) and can worsen the problem.[19]

High blood pressure, diabetes, thyroid disorders, and other health problems can cause vision loss also.

Newly blinded persons need to go through rehabilitation on an individual basis through a social service in their community, but then they must be allowed to try and take care of themselves. When this becomes impossible, a caregiver should step in. Caregivers should be aware of the services available for individuals who are visually handicapped or blind.

Services for those who are visually handicapped or blind are available in most cities. The services range from helping an individual get back into the job market to learning independent living skills. Many states list the services they offer in what are often called consumer guides to services for the blind and visually handicapped.

Services for the Blind and Visually Handicapped (SSB) is a subagency of a state's Department of Jobs and Training. Funded by state and federal dollars, SSB will not discriminate against anyone who may not be able to afford special equipment needed due to the disability.

Eligibility for SSB requires a visual disability that creates a major handicap and that the services will assist in rehabilitation. A visual handicap includes one of the following (as listed in the *Consumer Guide to Minnesota Services for the Blind and Visually Handicapped* [p. 9]):

1. 20/60 or less corrected central vision in the better eye with best correction;

2. a loss of one full quadrant of binocular field vision; or

3. a progressive eye condition which is likely to result in legal blindness (20/200 or less central vision in the better eye with best correction or side vision of less than 20 degrees).

An examination by a qualified opthalmologist should determine if the criteria have been met.

"SSB believes that blindness should never stop a person from succeeding in obtaining a job, in training, or in any activity which reflects his or her personal interests." When individuals seek services from SSB, they are assigned to a counselor who designs a rehabilitation plan with them. This plan is called the written plan, and services are provided until the written plan is fulfilled. The plan includes anything that helps the individual obtain skills to maintain a life without sight. Listed below are many services and programs available to which a caregiver may refer.

SERVICES

(as listed in *The Consumer Guide to Minnesota Services for the Blind and Visually Handicapped,* pp. 16–20)

Adjustment to Blindness

Counseling and training to teach alternate ways of doing such things as traveling, reading, taking notes and messages, and general home and self-management. This service ranges from a full-time program at a residential center to a part-time program in the home. Centers exist in many states and each individual can decide if this is a service he or she may be interested in.

Advocacy

Assistance in getting services from other agencies.

Business Enterprise Program

Specialized training to operate a vending facility such as a cafeteria, a snack bar, of a vending-machine enterprise.

Communication Center

Transcription of materials into Braille and onto tape. Cassette players, talking book machines, and Radio Talking Book Receivers are available at no charge to listen to materials produced by or available from the Communication Center.

Diagnostic Evaluation

Exams and other services for the visually handicapped person and his or her counselor to determine eligibility for services, design a rehabilitation goal, and to work toward the written plan.

Interpreter

The manual or tactile giving of oral or written communication to a deaf client so that clients can benefit from other services.

Job Placement

Leads on job openings, job market trends, job-seeking-skills training, and assistance to employers.

Low Vision

Services to help use or improve the use of existing vision to achieve the goal under the written plan.

Maintenance

Assistance in meeting basic living expenses, like housing and food, that result from getting services under the written plan.

Notetaking

Recording in Braille or the writing of notes, lectures, or meetings a client attends. This service must be needed so that the visually impaired individual can benefit from another service, such as vocational training.

Occupational Licenses, Tools, Equipment, or Initial Stocks and Supplies

Items needed for jobs such as machinist or a repair person or to be self-employed.

Orientation and Mobility

Training to travel safely and independently without sight.

**Other Goods and Supplies Related to
Employment or Vocational Training**

Any other service not listed here but needed by visually handicapped individuals to reach their goals.

Post-Employment Services

Assistance provided after a job is obtained so that visually handicapped individuals can keep their jobs or regain other suitable employment.

Reader Service

The oral reading of material needed to benefit from another service. The reading of a computer manual that is part of a training program is an example of how a reader service could be helpful in reaching a goal. The reading of the manual would occur if it were not available in Braille, on tape, or in large print.

Referrals

Assistance in locating and contacting other needed services.

Rehabilitation Counseling

Assistance in developing a positive attitude toward blindness and in moving toward personal and vocational independence.

Rehabilitation Engineering

The application of technologies, engineering methodologies, or scientific principles to meet the needs of and address barriers confronted by visually handicapped individuals in such areas as education, employment, transportation, and independent living that impact on their goals.

Rehabilitation Teaching

Instruction in performing things like homemaking and self-care activities without sight. This includes Braille reading and writing.

Restoration Services

Medical services meant to correct or improve physical conditions causing visually handicapped persons substantial problems. An example of a restoration service for some clients may be cataract surgery.

Services to Family Members

Needed assistance to a member of a client's family so the client can achieve his or her rehabilitation goal.

Telecommunication and Sensory Aids

Electronic equipment that improves or takes the place of one sense in a person. These aids also help overcome problems people have with walking or muscle control. A voice-output attachment on a computer is an example of a sensory aid that might be appropriate for some clients.

Transportation

Assistance provided to a visually impaired individual in order to get from one place to another to carry out the rehabilitation plan.

Vocational Training

Training at a college, vocational institute, or trade school. Services for the Blind will pay tuition only to the level charged at state universities, regardless of the program attended.

PROGRAMS

(as listed in the *Consumer Guide to Minnesota Services for the Blind,* pp. 21–27)

Vocational Rehabilitation Program

This program's goal is to have people obtain employment. Vocational testing is available, to learn more about the person's abilities and interests. Many of the services are available to help the individual reach the goal of obtaining employment.

Independent Living Program

The Independent Living Program helps people gain independence in their homes and in the community. The clients learn how to move about their homes with a cane, prepare meals, and perform self-care. There must be severe limitation in two or more of the following areas to be eligible: communication, travel, meal preparation, and self-care.

Self-Care Program

The Self-Care Program is available to people over the age of fifty-five who are likely to benefit from the services. This program includes services needed for the blind or visually handicapped to be able to take care of themselves. Most services in the above list will fit into this category.

CASE STUDIES

Mr. Parker is a very independent man of eighty-five and accustomed to driving himself about. His vision has deteriorated so much that he did not see a car moving toward him while he was at a stop sign. Mr. Parker pulled out into the road and the oncoming car crashed into the side of his vehicle. Luckily nobody was hurt in the accident, but now Mr. Parker is unable to renew his driver's license due to his poor vision. He feels trapped in his home and terribly dependent on his adult children, friends, and willing neighbors to drive him where he needs to go.

Driving can become very difficult because the ability to detect moving objects deteriorates.[20] This could pose a threat not only to elders, but to others who share the road with them. Caregivers should understand the depression an elder may feel when the independence of driving is taken away. Providing transportation for the elder should be incorporated into a caregiver's responsibilities.

Mr. and Mrs. Johnson, a couple married for fifty years, live in an apartment on their own. Mrs. Johnson usually does the cooking for both of them. One evening the Johnsons sat down to a meal of soup and sandwiches. Mr. Johnson tasted the soup first and proceeded to spit it out. As Mrs. Johnson wondered why he had behaved so rudely, she smelled what she thought was soup and realized that it was condensed milk. She did not tell her husband that her eyes had been failing her lately. Mr. Johnson felt terrible for his wife, but his eyes were not much better.

Making a meal, washing the dishes, reading food labels, or just reading a magazine may become impossible for some elderly people. Malnutrition may well be a reality for those elders who cannot drive to the grocery store, read the food labels, or see well enough to prepare a meal. Caregivers should be well-informed in the area of nutrition, so they can prepare meals for older adults who cannot do it themselves. Possibly, a caregiver could reteach a newly blinded individual how to prepare a meal. Many foods can be identified by touch and smell.

Ms. Reed had gone nearly blind in the last ten years due to macular degeneration. She has lived on her own for the last twenty years since her husband died. Lately, her favorite pastime, gardening, has become difficult. Ms. Reed still maintains a large garden and provides many fresh vegetables for her neighbors. Jackie, Ms. Reed's only daughter, lives a few hours away and visits at least once a month. Whenever Jackie is visiting, she does not let her mother lift a finger. Ms. Reed feels very useless and thinks her daughter lacks confidence in her.

Family members, friends, service providers, and casual contacts attempt to place a person with new vision loss in a sort of protective cocoon.[21] The sighted community needs to become educated to reverse the labeling process of the blind. It is important for visually impaired individuals to be allowed to perform as many activities as possible for themselves. A sense of accomplishment and a feeling of being needed are important to everyone, including those with impaired vision.

*　　*　　*

Mrs. Wegner, a woman of eighty-one, enjoys reading just about any kind of magazine and watching television. Lately, she has been constantly cleaning her reading glasses, but they do not seem to come clean. She sees a kind of whitish haze while reading. Upon visiting her doctor, she found out she has cataracts.

A possible solution for people with deteriorating vision could be to install better lighting in their homes. For a cataract sufferer, the light must not be too bright, because the brigher the light the more it tends to scatter, like bright light shining through dirty glass.[22] On bright sunny days, closing shades or blinds partially may help this person see better. Also, cataract surgery is a very viable answer these days.

Mrs. Hanson, a lady of eighty-one living in an assisted care apartment building, cannot see well enough to check her watch for the time. Mrs. Hanson ordered a special sensory aid: a watch that talks and can tell her the time by pushing a bar on the watch face. A local electronics store agreed to program the watches for anyone interested in them.

Specialty shops carry many sensory aids, anything necessary for the well-being and independent living of visually handicapped individuals. A few examples are white canes, playing cards in Braille, ice grippers to go over the shoes for traction in the winter, talking clocks and calculators, Braille or large-face watches, and adaptive cooking and sewing aids.

Mrs. Hanson is also very interested in current issues, but cannot read the newspaper. She had been an avid reader before the loss of her vision. Communication services are also available through Services for the Blind. Closed-circuit radios are available; these radios provide news, service announcements, the reading of magazines, newspapers, bestselling books, and even the reading of comic strips on Sunday mornings. Also available are books on tape, phonograph and tape players, Braille books, vocational and textbook material on tape or in Braille, library information on blindness, and repair services for the materials.

Mr. Dewey has enjoyed cooking all his life, especially when his large family comes to visit. He even dabbles in the art of gourmet cooking. Reading the special ingredients on the recipe cards that he traded with his gourmet cooking group has become difficult, due to the deterioration of his vision.

A solution to this problem is the printing of cookbooks in large print. A group called "The Adjustment to Blindness Partnership," has accomplished this task. The group compiled a cookbook of their favorite recipes and printed it in very large print.

*   *   *

Mr. Belfry, a seventy-five-year-old man living alone, has had the need for increasingly stronger prescription glasses every five years or so. He has been diagnosed with presbyopia and has the need for bifocals in his already quite high-power prescription glasses. Mr. Belfry worries that glasses will be very heavy and hurt his face.

A solution to this problem could be purchasing glasses made of a high-index plastic, able to provide for high-power prescriptions in a thin, light-weight plastic.

Listed below are some warning signs that an eye problem may exist, as listed in the October 1988 issue of *USA Today*. Elders and their caregivers should be aware of these warning signs.

1. Sudden hazy or blurred vision

2. Recurrent pain in or around the eyes

3. Double vision

4. Flashes of light or showers of black spots

5. Changes in color of the iris

6. Halos or rainbows around light

7. A dark spot at the center of viewing

8. Vertical lines look distorted or wavy

9. Excess tearing or "watery eyes"

10. Dry eyes with itching or burning.

All of these normal age-related changes in the eyes can make everyday tasks more difficult. Elders experiencing any of these symptoms should consult an opthalmologist or vision specialist for appropriate treatment.

Below are some tips for elders and caregivers.

1. Have your eyes checked at least every two years.

2. Know the common eye problems that occur with aging.

3. Know the warning signs of a possible eye problem.

4. Increase the amount of light for reading, sewing, and other close-up activities. For example, use a 100-watt bulb instead of a 60-watt bulb.[23]

5. "Watch TV from a distance of at least five times the width of the screen. For example, view a 19-inch screen from a distance of eight feet."[24]

6. Perform eye exercises three times a week. Some eye strain can possibly be alleviated and coordination improved with the help of a good exercise program. One such exercise could be moving the eyes up and down and side to side as far as one can.

Also, clocks and calendars with big print should be put around the house. Throw rugs or other loose objects on the floor should be removed. Reduced vision makes it difficult to see obstacles in one's path. Older adults are at a high risk of breaking a bone, should they happen to fall, and recovery from an injury due to a fall is a long, slow process.

New vision loss or blindness can be quite a difficult adjustment for elders living on their own. These people are at risk of doing damage to themselves as they perform everyday tasks. Family, friends, and caregivers should be available if these elders are not able to perform the tasks themselves.

NOTES

1. *USA Today,* "Growing Older with Good Vision," (October 1988).

2. Stephen C. Ainlay, "Aging and New Vision Loss: Disruptions of the Here and Now," *Journal of Social Issues* 44 (1988): 79–94.

3. Keith P. Bowen, "Aging Eyeballs," *Sky and Telescope* 82 (1991): 254.

4. Karen B. Clay, "Good Health: Eyes," *Essence Magazine* 21 (1991): 46.

5. Ainlay, "Aging and New Vision Loss: Disruptions of the Here and Now," and Donald Kline, "Treating Visual Aging," *USA Today* 113 (1985): 9–10.

6. Clay, "Good Health: Eyes."

7. *USA Today,* "Growing Older with Good Vision."

8. Bowen, "Aging Eyeballs."

9. *USA Today,* "Growing Older with Good Vision."

10. *USA Today,* "The Eyes: New Diagnostic Treatment for Glaucoma" (February, 1984): 113–19.

11. Bowen, "Aging Eyeballs."

12. *USA Today,* "The Eyes: New Diagnostic Treatment for Glaucoma."

13. Ibid.

14. *USA Today,* "Growing Older with Good Vision."

15. Bowen, "Aging Eyeballs."

16. Ibid.

17. Ibid.

18. Clay, "Good Health: Eyes."

19. Ibid.

20. Kline, "Treating Visual Aging."

21. Ainlay, "Aging and New Vision Loss: Disruptions of the Here and Now."

22. Karen Hahn, "Think Twice . . . About Sensory Loss," *Nursing* 19 (1989): 97–99.

23. Clay, "Good Health: Eyes."

24. Ibid.

ADDITIONAL REFERENCES

Consumer Guide to Minnesota Services for the Blind and Visually Handicapped. Compiled by the Minnesota Department of Jobs and Training (February 1990).

Jaques, Paul F. ". . . And the Risk of Developing Cataracts," *Science News* (1990): 137, 189.

6

Coping with Hearing Loss

Jennifer Remer

Aging is a natural process that all of us undergo. The physical changes of aging are inevitable in every part of the body. Cells that make up every organ begin to show the effects of aging as the cells stop reproducing. As people age, cell loss occurs in each organ, but each organ loses cells at a different rate.[1]

Often the biggest change that occurs during the aging process—the one that most people fear—is the loss of hearing. It is estimated that 75 percent of the people who reach eighty years of age have hearing impairments.[2] For many older people, the loss of hearing could mean the loss of communication. This causes great concern in elders. Understanding what causes the loss of hearing and how it can be prevented becomes very important to an elder's ability to communicate.

The loss of hearing can range from losing the ability to hear specific sounds, to complete silence. Losing the ability to hear only certain sounds can be very frustrating. Messages are misunderstood because an elder will hear only a portion of the message. Sometimes communication becomes as upsetting for the person doing the talking as it is for the elder who cannot hear well. Messages are repeated to the point that the elder, or the person speaking, may just give up.

The medical term *presbycusis* means a slow progressive loss of hearing due to nerve or bone damage of the inner, middle, or external ear. Loss of hearing, or deafness, can be caused by a number of things, from hardening of the arteries to stiffening of the joints in between the three bones of the ear.[3]

THE EXTERNAL EAR

The external ear, which is any part of the ear that can be seen or touched, is shaped specifically for picking up sound waves or vibrations and sending them to the ear canal. The ear canal leads to the eardrum, a thin membrane that closes off the ear canal. When a sound wave is channelled down the ear canal to the eardrum, it vibrates thereby causing the three ear bones located in the middle ear to vibrate. These three bones are joined together and the vibration moves from one bone to another until it reaches the inner ear, where the sound impulse is detected by the auditory nerve. The auditory nerve sends the message to the brain, where it is interpreted.[4]

EXTERNAL EAR PROBLEMS

If the ear canal is blocked off or obstructed, the sound wave will not reach the middle or inner ear where sound is detected. There are certain frequent problems that occur in the external ear that cause an impairment or loss of hearing: inflamed or swollen tissue in the ear canal and the buildup of ear wax or dust, which blocks off or obstructs the ear canal.[5] If there is a problem in the external ear, it may interrupt sound waves, causing the eardrum to vibrate differently or not to vibrate at all (if the sound waves are blocked off). When the eardrum picks up only part of a sound wave, an elder will not be able to interpret the sound. When either of these conditions occurs and the sound wave does not reach the eardrum, nothing will be heard or even detected, leaving the elder unaware that any message was sent.[6]

External Ear Infection

An external ear infection can cause a loss of hearing, too. The ear canal becomes inflamed, which results in painful swelling and sometimes draining of pus, either of which can partially or completely block the ear canal. An external ear infection can be caused by a number of factors. Swimming in water often forces bacteria into the ear canal causing an infection. Infection can also result from efforts to clean the ears. It is important to be careful when inserting a cotton swab into the ear canal because oftentimes it may be placed too deeply or pushed too hard into the ear. If the swab is pushed too hard or extends too far into the ear canal, it can cause ear wax to become packed, or it can scrape the tissue in the ear canal, causing an infection.[7]

Case Study

It was the Fourth of July, the sun was hot, the beach was crowded, and Grandpa James took his five grandchildren to the beach to cool off and enjoy the pleasures of summer. That Wednesday Grandpa James and his five grandchildren spent the entire day in cool lake water.

Grandpa James put on quite a show, performing swan dives and belly flops for his grandchildren. They were very impressed when they dared Grandpa James to dive all the way down to the bottom of the lake, and he brought up mud from the bottom to prove he could do it. But they were really impressed when Grandpa James performed his grand finale by playing "the hero of the lake," and swimming out to the middle of the lake to save a beach ball.

The following morning, after he awoke, James noticed that thick, yellowish-white fluid was draining from his ears. As James started to touch his ear with a tissue to dry it, he felt pain and tenderness around the opening of the ear. James got out of bed and walked into the bathroom to examine his ear in the mirror. The only thing that he noticed was the dark red color around the opening of the ear canal and the fluid that was draining out of it. The pain started to get worse the more he touched his ear, so he went to the clinic to be examined by a physician.

The doctor looked inside James's ear and told him that he had an external ear infection. James asked how his ear could have become so infected, and the physician listed a number of factors that cause the infection. James figured out that his ear infection was caused by swimming in the lake.

Ways to Avoid External Ear Infections

- Wear ear plugs when swimming.
- Do not place foreign objects into your ears.
- Clean your ears regularly.
- Gently clean your ears with a cotton swab, using a circular motion around the side of the canal.

Treatment for External Ear Infections

If an ear infection does occur, treatment is available. There are a number of antibiotics, solutions, and pain killers that can be prescribed by a doctor, so the loss of hearing caused by an external infection is not a permanent condition. However, it has been found that people who have suffered from such infections are more susceptible to external ear infections in the future.[8]

THE MIDDLE EAR

The middle ear is an air-filled cavity that lies behind the eardrum and consists of three tiny bones: the anvil, the hammer, and the stirrup. These three bones vibrate through a chain effect that starts with sound waves entering the ear, causing the eardrum to vibrate. The eardrum then pushes against the hammer, which is connected to the anvil, and sends the vibration along to the stirrup. Once the vibration reaches the base of the stirrup, it is transmitted through the temporal bone. The vibrations are sent through an opening of the temporal bone called an oval window. The vibrations are sent through this opening to the auditory nerve, where the "sound" is translated by the brain.[9]

PROBLEMS WITH THE MIDDLE EAR

The most common problem that occurs in the middle ear is the stiffening of the joints among the three ear bones and between the base of the stirrup and the oval window. Deafness or loss of hearing because of the inability of sound waves to be conducted to the brain is a condition called *functional deafness* or *conduction deafness*.[10] When the ear bones become diseased, the bones acquire a stickiness and pass a continued message to the auditory nerve. The result is a constant buzzing in the ears, which is called *otosclerosis*. The less external noise is present, the louder the buzzing sound seems. When there is little or no external noise—for example, before falling asleep—otosclerosis sounds like a loud, roaring noise. When in public places with a great deal of external noise, otosclerosis sounds like a quiet ringing.[11]

Treatment for Otosclerosis

The cause of otosclerosis is unknown, but it is possible that the condition could be hereditary. Due to the lack of information about this disease, the only treatment for otosclerosis is surgery to free the bones and restore normal vibration in the ear bones.[12]

THE INNER EAR

There are specific parts of the inner ear that are important for functions such as balance control, the transmission of sound waves, and the deciphering of sound waves into intelligible messages. The parts of the inner ear that are responsible for these functions are the semicircular canals, which control balance; the cochlea, which transmits sound waves; and the auditory nerve, which is responsible for the deciphering of sound waves.

THE SEMICIRCULAR CANALS

The semicircular canals consist of three canals placed at ninety-degree angles to each other and containing a fluid called *perilymph,* which moves around in the semicircular canals every time the body is in motion, like water moves around in a glass. Once the head is tilted or spun around, the perilymph moves, which allows for recognition of body position. The brain then detects the change in body position and makes the necessary muscular adjustments to maintain balance.[13]

PROBLEMS OCCURRING IN THE SEMICIRCULAR CANALS

When an inner infection occurs in the semicircular canals, *labyrinthitis* (inflammation of the inner ear) results. When the semicircular canals become irritated or infected, the motion of the fluid is exaggerated in its impulse to the brain, causing a spinning, unsteady sensation or a dizziness called *vertigo,* which is a whirling sensation. The more severe the labyrinthitis, the more difficult it becomes to control one's balance. The loss of balance may be so great that getting out of bed or out of a chair may become impossible.[14]

CAUSES OF AND TREATMENT FOR
SEMICIRCULAR CANAL PROBLEMS

Viral infections are the most common cause for semicircular canal problems, or labyrinthitis. It may take up to eight weeks before the infection clears up. During this time an elder will have problems with balance, and may suffer from recurring dizziness.[15]

Effective treatment can be prescribed by a physician who can identify this disease. The loss of balance and continual dizziness can be a frightening experience to an elder. When symptoms like these occur, the elder's physician should be consulted. Antihistamines are often prescribed by doctors to treat labyrinthitis; to reduce the symptoms of dizziness and the loss of balance.[16]

PROBLEMS THAT OCCUR WITH THE AUDITORY NERVE

The progressive loss of hearing, or *presbycusis,* directly affects the elder's ability to sense incoming sound. The loss of this ability occurs because, as a person ages, the arteries harden. When this happens, the blood supply to many parts of the body, including the ears, is reduced. One of the main parts of the ear where the blood supply is reduced is the auditory nerve. When incoming sounds are not heard correctly, or even detected, communication becomes very difficult. This means that certain sounds cannot be heard, such as high-pitched sounds. Signs of this type of hearing damage can be detected when words containing relatively high-pitched sounds are not recognized or are misinterpreted. There are certain high-pitched consonants that many elderly cannot hear: the sounds made to produce the letters s, f, p, t, k, ch, sh, and st are often not sensed by an elder with presbycusis damage. This causes misunderstanding because the elder is hearing only part of what is being said.[17]

CASE STUDY

"Dad, Sherry and I are heading up to Lake Superior this week to . . ." Cut off sharply by his father, David stops talking and waits patiently.

"Who's Harry?" his father questioned, after misinterpreting what his son had just said.

"Sherry, my wife." David stressed the "sh" on Sherry so his father could hear it.

But David's father thought his son misunderstood what he said by telling him his wife is Sherry and still wanted to know about Harry. "Yeah, I know Sherry's your wife. But who's Harry?" David's father insisted.

David, now aware that his father is really having a hard time hearing the message correctly, talks louder and really starts to move his mouth. David replies slowly, "No, Dad, "I'm going camping with Sherry, my wife, not Harry."

David's father, now realizing he misinterpreted the message, responds with, "Oh, so where did you say you were going?"

"We're going to Lake Superior," David happily replies now that his father is finally catching on.

Then his father says, "Lake Seerer. Never heard of it. Where is it?"

David rolls his eyes and starts to talk really slow, overemphasizing his syllables, "Lake S-U-P-E-R-I-O-R. Not Seerer, SUPERIOR. The Great Lake up north by Canada."

David's father, once again embarrassed and hurt because he cannot hear, replies with, "Oh, Lake Superior. This week you're going up there?" Tired of feeling stupid because he cannot hear, David's father seeks simple yes or no questions to save himself the embarrassment.

David answers with, "Yeah, we're planning on taking off after church."

David's father, not expecting anything more than a yes or no, answers with, "You're what?"

David, now sick of repeating everything he says, quickly repeats, "We're leaving after church."

Completely missing everything David said, his father asks, "You're leaving when?"

David rephrases his answer hoping his father will understand. "After mass this Sunday."

"O.K.," David's father replies.

David, not sure his father really heard him, repeats when he is leaving once again and keeps on talking without taking a breath, so his father cannot get a word in the conversation. "Yes, we are leaving after mass and we will be back next Monday, so is it possible that you and Mom could check the house, and make sure everything's O.K.?"

David's father, now very frustrated, repeats what he thinks he just heard, "You want Mom and I to keep an eye on the homestead?"

David, very happy that he got through to his father quickly, replies with a smile, "Yes, we'd really appreciate it; it would make us feel a lot more secure."

David's father smiles back but has no idea what his son just said: "What did you say?"

WAYS TO IMPROVE COMMUNICATION WITH AN ELDER WHO IS SUFFERING FROM A LOSS OF HEARING

- Look at the elder when you speak.
- Move your mouth to form each syllable carefully.
- Speak clearly.
- Use body language: act out what you are saying.
- Speak above a whisper.
- Speak slowly.
- Listen to the elder.

TREATMENT FOR AUDITORY NERVE DAMAGE

There is no known treatment for nerve damage. A hearing aid can help an elder to hear only if partial nerve damage has taken place. Even though the ability to hear cannot be restored to those with complete nerve deafness, the ability to communicate is still possible through facial expressions, body language, and lip reading. Nonverbal communication through body language and lip reading has been used by every individual at one time or another. Speaking is not the only form of communication that exists.

COPING WITH AN ELDER WHO SUFFERS FROM A LOSS OF HEARING

Communication is an essential part of life. The progressive or sudden loss of the ability to hear is difficult to face, even though we take for granted how important hearing is in everyday life. When an elder's ability to hear lessens, it is vital to realize what a special capacity the elder is beginning to lose. When an elder has had the ability to hear, and that ability becomes threatened by hardening of the arteries and the stiffening of joints, the older person at that point begins to realize what an important function hearing plays in life. Caregivers must realize that an elder is losing one of the most important elements of communication, namely, the ability to listen. Without the ability to hear what other people are saying, an elder may find it impossible to communicate. But communication must be sought in different ways if elders and those who care about them desire to make life as enjoyable and rewarding as possible.

NOTES

1. Barbara Silverstone and Helen Kandel Hyman, *You and Your Parents* (New York: Pantheon Books, 1989), p. 64.

2. Nora S. Ernst and Hilda R. Glazer-Waldman, *The Aged Patient* (Chicago: Year Book Medical Publishers, 1983), p. 147.

3. Robert Taylor, *Feeling Alive After 65* (New Rochelle, N.Y.: Arlington House Publishers, 1973), p. 40.

4. Ibid., pp. 39–40.

5. Silverstone and Hyman, *You and Your Aging Parents,* p. 303.

6. James Lally, *The Over 50 Health Manual* (Englewood Cliffs, N.J.: Prentice-Hall, 1961), p. 43.

7. Taylor, *Feeling Alive After 65,* p. 41.

8. Ibid., pp. 41–42.

9. Ibid., p. 40.

10. Mary Falconer, Michael Altamura, and Helen Duncan Behnke, *Aging Patients* (New York: Springer Publishing Company, 1976), p. 147.

11. Lally, *The Over 50 Health Manual,* pp. 42–43.

12. Taylor, *Feeling Alive After 65,* p. 40.

13. Lally, *The Over 50 Health Manual,* p. 45.

14. Taylor, *Feeling Alive After 65,* pp. 42–43.

15. Ibid., p. 43.

16. Lally, *The Over 50 Health Manual,* p. 45.

17. Ernst and Glaser-Waldman, *The Aged Patient,* p. 147.

7

Coping with Mobility Loss

Jennifer Remer

As the body ages, many changes occur that can cause a lack of mobility. When mobility decreases, daily functions may become difficult or even impossible. Losing the ability to perform daily functions becomes a great risk for someone who lives alone. Simple daily activities—walking, dressing, and writing—can be greatly affected by the decreased ability to move.

THE INEVITABLE ARTHRITIS

Arthritis is one of the diseases that older people complain about most often. Aching pain in joints or throughout the entire body, whether it is severe or minor, can make life more frustrating and more complex.[1] There is no one cause for the changes that occur in the joints of an older person, though arthritis is one of the most common chronic diseases that affect them. There are many types of arthritis. Two very common forms that afflict the elderly are *osteoarthritis* and *acute infectious arthritis*. The causes of arthritis can range from an infection, sprain, or fracture, to gradual degeneration of the joints.[2] Arthritis is caused by events that people cannot avoid, thus making it impossible to prevent.

OSTEOARTHRITIS

Osteoarthritis, which is the gradual degeneration of the joint, is most common in the elderly.[3] The joints that commonly become infected are those we use most often: those found in the hand, the wrist, the feet, and the knees.[4] Since these joints are used so often, it is important that they be fully mobile. If there is a loss of function in foot, hand, or wrist joints, everyday functions may become very difficult if not impossible to perform. Without the function of the wrist joint, elders may be unable to write, tie their shoes, or bathe. No longer having the ability to perform these daily tasks can become frustrating and even frightening to those afflicted with arthritis. Not only are they suffering from the pain of sore and stiff joints, they also suffer great disability from this disease.

People who live alone may find arthritis to be a threat to the lifestyle they have chosen. If the disease continues to spread, mobility gradually decreases. Osteoarthritis causes the joints to swell and stiffen, resulting in pain to the area affected. Odd as it may sound, pain can be a friend because it helps keep an elder from overusing the joint, yet maintaining mobility is essential. In the beginning stages of osteo-arthritis, the pain may keep those afflicted from actively moving the affected body part.[5]

CASE STUDY

Early in the month of September, when it came time to harvest, Ray started to notice a slight swelling around the knuckles of his hands along with cramps that increased the more he used his hands. Ray had been farming for forty-five years and had never run into any sort of problems that interfered with his work, except for a few bumps and bruises. Nothing from his work had ever physically disabled him for an extended period of time. As a farmer, Ray needed the use of his hands to do everything from milking the cows to driving the tractor for many long hard hours of the day. When harvesting season began in the fall, Ray spent his entire day driving from one field to another bringing in his crops. Ray began to drive the tractor long into the night. The number of hours he had to drive the tractor had greatly increased and so had the cramps in his hand. By the time Ray was finished driving tractor at night, his knuckles were swollen to twice their normal size. Every night the pain got worse and the swelling took longer and longer to go down. After the harvesting was finished, Ray assumed the problem with his hands would clear up. Instead, as the weather grew cool and damp, Ray's condition grew worse. The pain increased to the point that he could no longer milk all the cows alone and needed to hire help full-time. Ray finally faced the fact that his arthritis was not going to go away.

ACUTE INFECTIOUS ARTHRITIS

The areas of the body that become affected with acute infectious arthritis are those we use continuously throughout the day. Because the body parts are in such great need it becomes impossible to get by without using the joints. The loss of mobility increases as the joint is used more and more. There is a possibility that the joints may become completely impaired because of the amount of stress placed upon them. Continued use of the joints may cause cartilage to wear away, leaving bone to rub against bone or other joints. This causes a great deal of pain and limits movement considerably. Medical attention is needed when arthritis reaches this point. The lack of movement becomes a problem while the risk of injury and the inability to perform daily tasks increases.[6]

Whenever arthritis shows signs of increasing pain or swelling, medical attention should be sought. Frequently, elders fall into the habit of making excuses for the increased pain and swelling and therefore never do get the affected area examined by a physician. An elder may feel that the doctor can do nothing for the problem. Many times there may be no medical attention needed, but if the signs of damaging arthritis are continuously overlooked, permanent impairment of the joint may occur. The risk of losing complete use of the joint can make it very difficult for an elder to live alone. The deterioration—ranging from partial impairment to complete loss of function—can be stopped or slowed with medical attention. Even if no damage is occurring in the joints, medication can be given to reduce the pain and swelling.

CASE STUDY

Joyce's arthritis came on very gradually, so gradually that she had been affected with arthritis for almost ten years before she was ever diagnosed. It started in her fingers as a very slight pain, to which she soon grew accustomed. She blamed the pain on the cold, damp weather, which is often when arthritis is at its worst. But she did nothing about it, since it did not seem to worsen. The pain felt the same from day to day, so Joyce found no need to worry.

Years later she noticed swelling in her wrists and increasing pain with the onset of cold weather. As the weather grew colder and more damp the pain in her wrists became acute. Joyce put up with the pain, blaming it this time on all the knitting and sewing she had done during the snowy season. By the time spring arrived, Joyce's pain had subsided and the swelling disappeared.

Once again she was back into the whole routine of her life, still ignoring the signs of arthritis when she would occasionally experience a period of painful swelling in her wrist and finger joints. She would apply ice packs to reduce the swelling and take aspirin to relieve the pain.

Joyce lived alone in a small white house ever since her husband passed away. She had many visitors, including her sons, daughters, neighbors, and friends who visited her a couple times a week. Joyce was very active, she took long walks, grew a huge garden, and loved to watch her grandchildren.

Joyce always managed to keep her occasional arthritic flare-ups to herself. Every winter when her arthritis started to affect her, the roads became covered with snow and ice, so visits were not as frequent. She became an expert at hiding the disability the arthritis caused; she would have everything ready when her guests arrived so she had little to do in their presence. But every year it took longer and longer for her to get ready for her guests.

One winter it started to take six or seven hours to get one meal ready for six people. Then one extremely cold, damp autumn her wrists and fingers swelled up bigger than they ever had before. She applied ice and took aspirin four or five times a day before she finally realized that this time she was suffering from something serious. It got to the point that she could no longer pick up a toothbrush or pencil. Getting dressed took hours and cooking became impossible.

This time the arthritis had become so disabling that she could do nothing but rock in her chair and take walks through the snow. Her wrists and fingers became so deformed that she could no longer use them. Finally, one snowy day the pain and swelling were so intense that she could make nothing to eat. This was when Joyce decided she could no longer live the way she had for the past month. She called the operator at 8:00 in the morning, unable to dial her daughter's phone number without pushing the wrong buttons.

Fifteen minutes later her daughter arrived at Joyce's house very concerned and surprised at her mother's condition. She embraced her mother before rushing her to the hospital.

STRUGGLING WITH THE INCREASING LOSS OF MOBILITY

As an elder strives for independence, it becomes very important that caregivers and friends recognize any increased loss of mobility. The gradual loss of mobility due to the stiffening of joints can make getting dressed, bathing, and cooking more difficult and painful with each passing day. There are ways caregivers and friends can assist without making an elder feel helpless. When getting dressed becomes a problem for an elderly person, the caregiver can buy clothes that can be easily changed: clothes without buttons, laces, or hooks. If cooking becomes a problem, the caregiver or friend can help by inviting the elder over to share a meal. One day could be set aside each week for the elder to dine with the caregiver, or the elder could be taken out occasionally to a favorite restaurant. Do not insist that the elder wear only a certain type of clothing; often it is easier to throw on a sweater than to button up a blouse. This can cause an elder to feel resentment and irritability toward the caregiver. If anybody knows how difficult these tasks can be, it is the elder. Elders do not want to be constantly reminded that it takes them longer to perform certain tasks than it did when they were younger. If anything, elders want to hear that they are improving, not getting worse. If elders suddenly feel that caregivers think the physical problems are going to take over the elders' lives, these older adults may become distant and avoid their caregivers for fear of no longer being in control of their own lives. Now more than ever before, it becomes very important that caregivers show care and, most of all, respect for these elders. Do not insult an older person's intelligence or capability by saying, "Do it this way, it's easier." Caregivers must work at being patient, thoughtful, and considerate.

Imagine how you would feel if someone took charge of your life and forgot about your feelings. Picture this situation when a daughter insists that her mother let her take her out or make dinner in order to make things easier for her mother.

CASE STUDY

"Mom, I noticed that you are having a hard time cooking lately, so why don't I take you out?"

The mother reacts by denying her daughter's statement and then making an excuse for the statement that is not supposed to be true: "I'm not having a hard time cooking. I'm fine. I've just been tired lately. I can cook just fine. I don't need to go out somewhere to eat. I can eat at home."

The daughter ignores her mother and continues to tell her that she will not be cooking tonight: "Well, if you don't want to go out, then I'll make you dinner."

The mother, becoming irritated, answers: "No."

The daughter continues to insist that she is right: "Mom, I know it would be easier on you if you went out or if I made you dinner."

Now frustrated, upset, and hurt that her daughter is not listening to her or showing her the respect that she needs and deserves, the mother demands that her daughter leave her alone: "I have heard enough. I wish that you would just let me live my own life the way I want to. If you really want to make my life easier, just leave me alone."

ADVICE ON HOW TO DEAL WITH THE LOSS OF MOBILITY

Just because the caretaker believes that doing something for the elder, like going out to eat or doing daily tasks, would make life easier physically, this generosity is by no means easier on an elder's state of mind. Doing daily tasks for an older person can increase the elder's feelings of helplessness and decrease self-esteem. It is difficult enough to face the idea that one can no longer perform daily tasks alone. The elder needs no reminders from caregiver, friends, or family. Caregivers should be concerned for elders' feelings. Offering to take an elder out means a great deal when the caregiver simply wants the older person's company, but not when it is thought that the elder should go out because he or she is getting older and suffers from a lack of confidence.

The best way to help elders is to show them friendship and love. The best feeling in the world is to feel wanted and loved, so give elders the love and caring that they need. A little appreciation can go a long way.

WARNING SIGNS OF ARTHRITIS

In situations where the joint's surface may be wearing down from the rubbing of bones or other joints, it is important to notice the signs of increased limitation and pain. When symptoms like this occur it could signal bone destruction or stiffening of the joint, both of which could lead to permanent impairment of the joint. Elders could lose complete function of their hands or feet if the situation is not treated. It is important to watch for signs of continued swelling and increased pain. When these symptoms appear for a prolonged period of time, or seem to have increased, medical attention is needed.

The Signs of Arthritis

- Increased swelling in the joints
- Increased pain
- Decreased mobility
- Reddening or yellowing of skin around joints
- The spread of symptoms to other joints.

If these signs appear, medication or other medical attention can clear up or help control the effects of arthritis.[7]

CHRONIC BACKACHE

Another problem that affects many people is chronic backache, which is believed to be the result of the aging process. Aching pain anywhere along the spine can cause immobility and can become a great risk to an elder who is home alone. When the back is injured or disabled, it becomes almost impossible to move any limbs of the body without causing further injury. If movement is possible, the pain that is radiated from the use of the back is so great that an elder may choose to not move at all. Failure to get up out of a chair because of back pain can make an elder feel helpless and weak. Nobody wants to feel like a burden as a result of not being able to perform as well as had been the case in the past. The loss of mobility that comes from chronic backache can cause an elder to become isolated at home for fear of not being able to move around independently. If an older person lacks the confidence to try to overcome or to find a cure for the backache, the condition could worsen to the point that the back could become deformed.[8]

SEVERE BACK PAIN

It is important to realize that the pain may need medical attention, but it is also important to know that minor back pain can often be relieved in ways that the elder can control. Some back discomfort can be caused by things as simple as a mattress that is too soft to be supportive for the back or by sleeping with the body out of alignment. When glasses do not fit properly elders sometimes move their heads in abnormal positions in order to see more clearly, thereby bringing about neck and back pain. Poor posture while sitting or standing can also be the reason for back pain.[9] A well-meaning caregiver or friend who continuously nags the elder to "sit up straight," probably accomplishes little beyond creating hard feelings. Instead, it should be mentioned that when elders sit down there is a tendency to slouch, and this could be a contributing factor in backaches. This approach will get much better results because most people are more receptive to gentle suggestions than to being ordered or bossed around.

Back pain in most cases can be treated. Time must be spent trying to find out what the likely cause could be. Many times, as in the case of poor posture, discovering and correcting the cause of the pain often ends in a satisfactory treatment.

RISKS OF CHRONIC BACKACHE

Helping older persons because they are having trouble becomes very important as the condition of elders worsens. Family members, friends, and caregivers may find it hard to know just how much help and guidance an elder needs. Often, those who wish to help go overboard and try to change the elder's lifestyle. This can cause the elder to withdraw and become isolated, creating an even worse problem.

Elders who suffer from chronic back pain should not be left alone at home or in bed for long periods of time. This can create both physical and psychological problems. The pain may become so intense some days that getting out of bed is impossible, but becoming bedridden for any period of time can cause additional problems. If older persons do not move their bodies while bedridden, continuous pressure on the unmoved body areas will restrict the blood supply. The lack of blood to any part of the body will cause skin ulcers or bed sores to form.

Now it becomes very important for caregivers to understand an elder's problems and special needs. The problems cannot be ignored, nor can the parties involved pretend that they will go away. Neglect will only cause the problems to get much worse. Often elders will act as if a problem is temporary and will just disappear, that one morning they will wake up and the problem will just be gone. In part this may be wishful thinking; then again, it may be an effort not to trouble caregivers, friends, and family. Instead of a miraculous recovery, the result of this ignorance and neglect may be a painful surprise.

FINDING A WAY TO DEAL WITH BACKACHE

When back pain is caused by bad habits and carelessness, the problem will not go away unless it is corrected. This takes time and effort from caregivers and the elders who are bearing the burden of back pain.

In some cases, the mind can be the source of the healing process. Confidence and self-esteem can lead to a positive state of mind that helps in the healing process. Elders need caregivers to help build their confidence, not to show pity toward them. Feeling sorry for elders is not going to give them the help or encouragement they need to correct the back problem. Caregivers should express positive and supportive feelings toward the elderly: this establishes an atmosphere of comfort in which elders are more likely to express their feelings and needs. This type of relationship will give the elderly the confidence needed to confront and overcome back pain.

When bad habits are not the cause of the back pain, or when the pain has reached the point that merely correcting the problem is not enough, medical attention is necessary. Aspirin and simple pain killers can be very helpful in relieving minor back pain, but oftentimes major back problems can only be corrected by surgery or other medical procedures. When no obvious solution can be found for an elder's back pain, a physician should be consulted.

Ways to Avoid Back Pain

- Never bend from the waist when lifting something.
- Never lift a heavy object without help.
- Avoid high-heel shoes.
- Sleep on a firm mattress.
- Do not slouch.
- Avoid prolonged standing.[10]

OSTEOPOROSIS

Through the aging process the bones begin to lose calcium, a mineral that is very important for their strength and endurance. When bone begins to lose calcium and mass, it becomes brittle and weak, making it easier to break. This condition is known as osteoporosis. An estimated twenty-four million people suffer from osteoporosis. The chances that an elder is suffering from this disease are very high. The cause of osteoporosis has not been found, but the deficiency of dietary calcium and metabolic imbalance have been associated with it.[11]

PROBLEMS RESULTING FROM OSTEOPOROSIS

With the resulting lack of bone mass, fractures can easily occur. It is no surprise that a higher percentage of broken bones and fractures occurs in the elderly. Because the number of pain receptors—the specific areas of the body that detect pain—decrease with age, an older person with broken bones or fractures may not feel the pain that a younger person would. Even though it may not cause an elderly person as much pain, a fractured or broken bone poses as much of a threat to those of advanced age as it would to anyone else. It should also be noted that the healing process slows down with age: many times a fracture may be more threatening to an older person since more time is needed for adequate healing to take place. When an older person is immobilized for an extended length of time due to a broken bone or fracture, the crippling effects of arthritis could occur because of the injured bone and the lack of mobility.

Accidents have become an increasingly important cause of death and disability among the elderly. This becomes a great risk to an elder living at home, since one-half of all accident fatalities occur in the home. It becomes an even greater risk if the elder suffers from osteoporosis. An accidental trip on a rug could end with a long stay in the hospital.[12]

CASE STUDY

One night, late in December, after a few inches of sticky wet snow had fallen, Mrs. Johnson drove to the grocery store to pick up a few things she needed to finish up her holiday baking for the Christmas cookie exchange that was being held the next day in the church basement. She only needed to buy a few items, which would have taken twenty minutes, but ended up taking more than an hour after she spent thirty minutes talking to Mrs. Davis and Mrs. Olson, who were both picking up items for the cookie exchange. Mrs. Johnson then spent another fifteen minutes visiting with the cashier, who was friends with her granddaughter, Melissa.

By the time Mrs. Johnson had finished shopping, it was dark, and the temperature had dropped considerably. It was late and there were only a few cars left in the parking lot. The cold wind blew in her face, causing her to shiver and walk quickly toward her car, which was parked next to an old pick-up truck. The parking lot was lighted only by the neon sign on the other side of the parking lot. As the wind blew harder, Mrs. Johnson started to speed up her walk as she approached the car. Suddenly, just a few feet away from her car, Mrs. Johnson stepped on a patch of ice. Sensing herself losing balance, she reached for the car to steady herself. Instead, she turned so quickly that her legs came out from under her and her groceries flew into the air as she fell to the ground. Mrs. Johnson landed on her right side with a crack. Her hip broke from the fall and her body ached. She tried to scream for help, but the shock from what had just happened kept her from being heard. Barely conscious, Mrs. Johnson lay in pain between her car and the old truck, unable to move. Two hours after her accident, she was discovered by the cashier and rushed to the hospital.

FEAR CAUSED BY OSTEOPOROSIS

This story may be very familiar, since there are an estimated 200,000 hip fractures in the United States each year.[13] Hip fractures are one of the most common fractures resulting from a fall. This fact causes elders to become terrified of falling. The fear of falling may result in elders staying away from activities they would normally perform. Confidence must be reestablished in older persons who fear falling. If this fear continues to grow, they may confine themselves to their homes. Emphasizing their strength and coordination can making elders feel more confident about themselves.

TREATMENT FOR OSTEOPOROSIS

There are thousands of ways to break a bone, but there are only a few ways to prevent bones from breaking in the first place. One way elders can increase the strength of their bones is to increase the amount of calcium taken on a daily basis. This can be done by diet or taking calcium supplements. Exercise also makes bones stronger and more durable. Both diet and exercise can improve bone strength, and can increase a person's overall mobility.

With increased strength and mobility elders will feel much more confident and capable. Exercising and eating right can give their bodies every possible advantage. Living carefully and wisely, but with confidence, can give elders the feeling of competence and success. With a bit of prevention, elders living alone need not live at risk.

Ways to Avoid Osteoporosis

- Eat a diet high in calcium.

- Take calcium pills or supplements if calcium in your diet is not adequate.

- Exercise at least three times a week.

WHAT TO DO IF THE PROBLEMS CONTINUE TO WORSEN

When elders suffer from arthritis, backache, or osteoporosis, any of these conditions may degenerate to the point where those afflicted can no longer function alone. When this occurs, older persons will often need to live with someone who can help. There are a number of apartment complexes that have a primary caregiver who will help with meals, bathing, dressing, and any other activities that need attention. The housing is set up so that the elders can continue to live as they wish but in safety. These individuals may not be able to do everything they once could, but they can do enough on their own so that skilled care facilities are not an option. This type of housing will allow the elder to live comfortably and safely.

WORDS OF ENCOURAGEMENT

As elders go through these changing times, caregivers, friends, and family must remember that help and encouragement are vital. Try to help only when asked, or ask first if the elder would like help. Try to be available for the elder as much as possible, and establish an atmosphere of mutual trust, so the older person feels that help will be there in time of need. It is very important to remember that elders need care and understanding from those who wish to help, and if they know it's there, it will make life much easier to manage and enjoy.

NOTES

1. Barbara Silverstone and Helen Kandel Hyman, *You and Your Parent* (New York: Pantheon, 1989), p. 327.

2. Mary W. Falconer, Michael V. Altamura, and Helen Duncan Behnke, *Aging Patients* (New York: Springer Publishing Company, 1976), pp. 98–100.

3. Silverstone and Hyman, *You and Your Parents*, p. 327.

4. Falconer, Altamura, and Behnke, *Aging Patients*, pp. 98–100.

5. James Lally, *The Over 50 Health Manual* (Englewood Cliffs, N.J.: Prentice-Hall Inc., 1961), p. 200.

6. Falconer, Altamura, and Behnke, *Aging Patients*, p. 98.

7. Ibid., pp. 98–100.

8. Lally, *The Over 50 Health Manual*, pp. 196–97.

9. Robert Taylor, *Feeling Alive After 65* (New Rochelle, New York: 1973), p. 127.

10. Ibid.

11. Silverstone and Hyman, *You and Your Parents*, pp. 331–32.

12. Nora Ernst and Hilda Glazer-Waldman, *The Aged Patient* (Chicago: Year Book Medical Publishers, 1983), pp. 105–106.

13. Ibid., p. 105.

8

How Elders Can Stay Active and Fit

Kenneth R. Ecker, Ph.D., and Paul M. Gordon, Ph.D., M.P.H.

INTRODUCTION

Concern over the steady rise in the cost of medical care in the United States has emerged as a principal issue that needs rectified in order to provide universal access to adequate healthcare. Good healthcare has become a luxury for some, while many find basic healthcare unaffordable. People over sixty-five, who rely mostly on public healthcare, have begun to question whether their medical coverage is adequate. Healthcare coverage in the elderly population has gained attention because of the demand this group places on the medical community. The elderly typically incur more medical expenses than younger age groups. This is further complicated by a burgeoning elderly population. A decrease in mortality rates over the years has increased life expectancy; more individuals are reaching their senior years. Moreover, the age of the population has changed dramatically. In 1950, there were 12.4 million elderly.[1] With the exploding birth rate following WW II, many of these individuals will approach retirement age within the early part of the next century. It has been estimated that by the year 2000 the elderly population is expected to swell to 35.4 million.[2] These estimates, in addition to increasing medical care costs, place the access to healthcare for the elderly in jeopardy. Health officials, realizing the seriousness of this problem, have set objectives for the year 2000 to minimize the demand the elderly place on medical care. Of primary importance is to improve the health span of the elderly, including those with chronic disease. Through lifestyle modifications preventive measures can be taken to promote self-reliance. Lifestyle interventions, such as habitual physical activity and good nutrition, are effective means of preventing disease and disability in the elderly, thus reducing their reliance on health care and, in particular, the need for long-term medical assistance.

The quality of life in the elderly can vary quite markedly. Extreme differences in the physical well-being and activity patterns of elderly individuals contributes to their ability to be self-sufficient. For many, approaching old age means becoming increasingly more dependent on others, often relying on nursing care or loved ones for even their basic needs. These elderly, who are not self-sufficient, often suffer from poor self-esteem and mental depression. On the contrary, preventive care, including regular exercise, can improve these situations. A daily exercise program can increase the range of independence among elderly individuals and reduce their reliance on healthcare. Moreover, those elderly with chronic disease who undertake habitual activity may reduce their reliance on others and improve their quality of life.

EXERCISE AND AGING

A lifetime can be divided into a growth and maturation period and an aging period. Since we study growth and development to implement physical education courses for school-age young people, it is reasonable that we be introduced to the aging theories as a prelude to implementing programs of physical activity for mature and aging individuals.

Obviously, aging is not an abrupt change in physiological functioning; it is a more gradual change occurring over several decades. Presently we do not understand the complete mechanisms of aging, nor do we understand how to reverse the aging process. However, aging and illness are not synonymous. Aging involves a gradual loss of functional capacity that may lessen the vigor and speed with which we do various activities, but it does not necessarily prevent us from doing them. Aging is universal, progressive, irreversible, and time-dependent: we cannot stop it, and it happens to everybody. But much of what we consider aging is not aging at all. Sometimes it is difficult to separate what is true nonpreventable aging from what is a result of changing lifestyles or acquired disability. For example, the decrease in physical fitness that is seen in many older people is, for the most part, the result of a decrease in physical activity, not aging per se.

AGE-RELATED CHANGES IN MUSCLE FUNCTION

Strength

Although we know of no definite threshold age for deterioration of performance, several performance criteria are altered (reduced in most cases) with aging. Most researchers have found that rapid improvement in strength accompanies the growth of children, and maximal strength is found to occur for most muscle groups between the ages of twenty-five and thirty.[3] Rodahl has shown that this increase in strength is due largely to the increased size of the muscle.[4] We should keep in mind that muscle strength is closely related to muscle cross-sectional area (the density of the long part of the muscle). The increase in cross-sectional area accounts for most of the gain in strength during growth and development.

Strength decreases very slowly during maturity. After about the fifth decade, strength decreases at a greater rate, but even at age sixty the loss does not usually exceed 10 to 20 percent of the maximum, with women's losses being somewhat greater than those of men.[5] The decrease in strength during aging can be partly accounted for by decreased muscle size, which is probably due to age-related alterations in the body's ability to synthesize protein. There is a loss of fibers from individual motor units within muscle tissue itself. This results in less available contractile force when this motor unit is recruited to stimulate muscle fibers to contract. Because of the decreases in both the size and number of muscle fibers within an individual muscle, this results in decreases in the muscle's respiratory capacity (its ability to use oxygen from the blood) as well as increases in fat and connective tissue. These changes can have severe consequences in the elderly: mobility may be hampered, incidents of soft tissue pain are more common, and the muscles' capacity to work is impaired. Aging results in decreased isometric and dynamic strength as well as speed of movement.[6]

The loss of the muscle's biochemical capacity is characterized by decreased activity of oxidative (oxygen using) and glycolytic (sugar using) enzymes, which are very important from a number of physiologic reasons, such as energy production and breakdown within the muscle.[7]

The mechanisms involved in muscle contraction are also impaired, which contributes to the loss of strength and power. Aging muscle has been found to be less excitable and, as a result, takes more time to complete it's contractile sequence. Thus, a greater stimulus is needed for contraction and a longer period of time is required before the muscle can respond to another stimulus.[8]

Capacity for Hypertrophy

Relative strength changes from training are similar in the young and the old, at least in short-term programs. Available research indicates a fundumental difference in the way old and young men gain strength through weight training. Young men increase strength primarily by increasing the muscle's size, whereas the old men (and young women) increase strength by increased neural stimulation).[9] Young and old men have demonstrated similar and significant percentage increases in strength, although the young have made greater absolute gains. Thus, the young improve the contractile capacity of the muscle fibers through more protein synthesis, while the elderly rely on improved motor unit recruitment. The diminished capacity for increasing muscle size in older males may also be related to decreased testosterone output. The hormone testosterone is important for protein uptake and synthesis by the muscle in order to maintain or increase muscle mass.[10]

Neural Function

Many neurophysiological changes occur with aging. Many times it is difficult to separate changes due to aging from those that occur with disease states. The principal changes include decreased visual acuity, decreased hearing ability, deterioration of short-term memory, inability to handle different types of incoming information simultaneously, and decreased reaction time.[11]

Recent research appears to suggest that a lifestyle of vigorous physical activity may have a beneficial effect in lessening the decline in reaction and movement times.[12] Spirduso has developed a mechanism to explain the relationship of exercise upon the nervous system based on similar research data portraying age effects and Parkinsonism.[13] A loss of brain cells that produce the neurotransmitter dopamine occurs both in normal aging and at an accelerated rate in Parkinsonism. Based on much of her work, Spirduso suggests that exercise may postpone the deterioration in reaction time, which generally happens in the aging nervous system, by maintaining the physiological integrity of the brain cells that produce dopamine. Because of her research in this area, she suggests that increased physical fitness may lessen the symptoms of aging by maintaining the physiologic function of the nervous system.[14]

Body Composition

It is readily apparent in a number of studies that with increasing age body fat increases in both sexes.[15] This should not be considered a normal trend, because other studies have shown that regular physical activity after age thirty-five can often inhibit any increase in body fat.

Increased body fat with age is of concern because of its possible relationship to many disease states (i.e., arthritis, gout, cancer, heart disease, etc.) as well as premature death. Exercise is extremely important in controlling body composition in the elderly. Metabolic rate slows with age, which necessitates a low-caloric diet in order to maintain weight and normal body composition. This decrease in overall body metabolism is caused mainly by a decrease in lean body mass, due to inactivity, along with an increase in body fat. The low-calorie diet of many older individuals is often low in many necessary vitamins and minerals. A regular exercise program would allow the elderly to consume more calories and also satisfy their nutritional requirements.[16]

By definition, obesity exists when fat tissue makes up a greater-than-normal fraction of total body weight. In male subjects aged eighteen, approximately 15 to 18 percent of body weight is fat.[17] The corresponding figure for females is 20 to 25 percent.[18] The percentage of body weight that is fat, as mentioned earlier, usually increases with age, but this is not always necessary or desirable. Obesity has been defined as a body fat content greater than 25 percent of the total body weight for men and greater than 30 percent for women.[19]

THE BENEFITS OF MOTION AND PHYSICAL ACTIVITY

Habitual exercise can be an effective means in both disease prevention and rehabilitation. Exercise impacts several chronic diseases including heart disease, stroke, diabetes, osteoporosis, certain cancers, low back pain, and mental health, to name a few. This list is not exhaustive by any means. In fact, researchers are repeatedly finding new means by which exercise is beneficial for disease prevention and rehabilitation. The following is a brief review of the role exercise plays regarding some of these chronic diseases.

Atherosclerosis

Atherosclerosis is the process whereby fats in the blood stream accumulate causing a narrowing in the affected arteries. This disease process can occur in the heart, brain, and legs. It is largely responsible for most of the heart disease, stroke, and clotting in the legs found in the general population. Physically active people have a lower risk for these diseases than those who are sedentary. Moreover, individuals with known disease who exercise under strict guidelines can reduce the progression of the disease. Exercise conditioning is effective at reducing risk for disease by modifying those variables which place individuals at risk. Among the risk factors for atherosclerotic disease that an exercise program can alter are: blood cholesterol, blood pressure, obesity, diabetes, and physical activity. For example, high levels of HDL cholesterol have been shown to reduce risk of heart disease.[20] Known as the good cholesterol, HDL is responsible for preventing a build up of fatty deposits within the blood stream. Individuals who undergo habitual physical activity have higher levels of HDL cholesterol. In combination with a low cholesterol/low saturated fat diet, exercise has even greater benefits. While dieting is an effective means of lowering total blood cholesterol, exercise maintains an elevated HDL cholesterol level. The result is a lower total cholesterol made up of a greater portion of HDL.

Another risk factor for heart disease is high blood pressure. Exercise has been shown to decrease mild hypertension. For many individuals, exercise prevents the need for medication therapy. Habitual physical activity can be effective in those who rely on blood pressure medications. Exercise can even help to reduce the reliance on such medications. Often the amount of medication must be reduced following exercise therapy.

Perhaps the greatest effect exercise therapy has on risk factor modification is through weight loss. Obesity is associated with increased risk for several diseases including heart disease, diabetes, and some cancers.[21] Physical activity increases the burning of calories, which is an effective means for weight loss. In fact, when exercise therapy complements dieting, weight loss is most productive. In addition, muscle deterioration is prevented when weight loss occurs as a result of a combined diet and exercise program. In contrast, when weight loss occurs from dieting alone, a portion of lean muscle tissue is lost. Nevertheless, when weight loss occurs, other risk factors are reduced. For example, losing weight can reduce blood pressure, lower cholesterol, and improve blood glucose (blood sugar) levels.

Research also suggests that lack of physical activity, in itself, is a risk factor for atherosclerotic disease. If you were to control for all risk factors except sedentary lifestyle, the risk of disease would be higher than in physically active individuals. The direct association of exercise on atherosclerotic risk is not fully understood. Certain clotting factors in the blood stream are modified in physically active individuals.[22] Also, habitual exercise enhances the pumping capacity of the heart. Subsequently, the efficiency of the heart is improved, which reduces the energy required for the heart to function. By reducing the amount of work the heart must do we may prevent or delay the atherosclerotic process.

The aging process naturally alters the function of the heart. For example, the ability of the heart muscle to contract decreases as a consequence of aging.[23] However, this process may be delayed or impeded through staying physically active. In general, individuals who continue to be physically active alter the overall rate of physical decline that occurs with aging.

The risk of atherosclerotic diseases, such as coronary artery disease and stroke, is markedly reduced through a risk factor modification program that includes exercise intervention. Furthermore, physical activity programming improves cardiovascular function, which prevents or delays the natural aging processes and enhances cardiovascular health.

Diabetes Mellitus

Adult onset diabetes can be characterized as a disease of aging. Often times adult onset or type II diabetes goes undetected until blood screenings (taken after a period of fasting) reveal an elevated glucose level. The long-term effects of uncontrolled diabetes can result in heart disease, blindness, kidney failure, and nerve disease. Habitual physical activity plays an important role in controlling blood glucose levels and improving the detrimental progression of this disease.

Type II diabetes is highly associated with obesity, meaning that individuals who are excessively overweight are at increased risk of contracting the disease. Weight loss is an effective means of controlling type II diabetes. In fact, as weight loss occurs, the diabetic symptoms typically improve. As previously mentioned, habitual exercise assists in weight reduction through the burning of calories. Overweight individuals who participate in a regular exercise program are more likely to reduce excess fat than through dietary regimens alone.

Exercise therapy is also effective in controlling blood glucose.

Normally, the hormone insulin, produced in the pancreas of a healthy individual, is responsible for clearing glucose from the blood stream. However, the insulin produced in type II diabetics is not effective at lowering blood glucose, often leaving the patient dependent on medications. Exercise has a natural insulin-like response, which assists in lowering glucose in the blood stream. Due to this response, a diabetic beginning an exercise program may be required to cut back on medication. Furthermore, in physically active people, insulin is more effective at lowering blood glucose than in persons who are inactive. Therefore, less insulin is needed to control glucose levels in the blood stream. For the diabetic who undergoes exercise therapy, improving the sensitivity of insulin further aids in reducing the need for medication.

Habitual activity is effective in the prevention and rehabilitation of type II diabetes. The aggregate effect of exercise therapy on diabetes is to improve the effectiveness of insulin produced in the body and promote weight control, which reduces the reliance on medications to control blood glucose.

Osteoporosis

At present, population demographics have revealed an aging population.[24] As a process of aging, the structure of the skeletal bones changes. The mineral content of the bone can become depleted, leaving poris or brittle bone (*osteoporosis*). The mineral content begins to decline at approximately thirty-five to forty years for both men and women. In women, loss of bone mass increases to 2 to 3 percent per year after menopause.[25] Men lose bone mineral at a rate of .3 to .5 percent per year.[26] The risk for developing osteoporosis can be attributed to inadequate calcium intake, depleted estrogen hormones, and decreased physical activity. Consequently, osteoporosis is more likely to affect post-menopausal women. Because of this, elderly women are at greater risk than elder men. However, elderly men who are advanced in age can be at comparable risk. Depleted bone mass resulting from osteoporosis increases the likelihood of skeletal fractures, which can be difficult to heal. Individuals are often left disabled making it impossible for them to perform simple daily activities. The loss of bone mass can be prevented or minimized through a combined regimen of diet and exercise. Increased calcium intake is recommended to replenish the loss of bone calcium that occurs in hormone depleted individuals. However, increased calcium intake does little to offset the loss of bone mineral if physical activity is not included.

Aside from the benefits of increased muscular strength and endurance derived through the appropriate programs, bones generally adapt quite well to the stress that exercise places on them. In general, habitual exercise can increase bone mass in young individuals and improve or retard loss in older patients. Studies of tennis players reflect this well. Since tennis players subject one arm (their racquet arm) to much more stress than the other, their arm bones can be compared to illustrate this difference as it relates to exercise. In a study of professional tennis players, the dominant arm or racquet arm showed a greater thickness in the upper arm bone by 25 percent in comparison to the nondominant arm. Even in elderly groups of tennis players who play only several hours a week (8 hours approximately) the upper arm bone was 4 percent wider in the dominant arm and had 13 percent more mineral per centimeter of bone. These differences were much greater than was observed in sedentary players of the same age.[27]

Improvements in bone mass more commonly occur in joints that are physically stressed. For example, an habitual walking program is more likely to improve bone mass in the back, legs, and feet. However, improvements would not likely occur in the arms. For this reason, muscle strengthening programs, which can incorporate the total body, are effective. Activities that place gravitational stress on the bones, such as walking, jogging, tennis, and resistive training are helpful for maintaining bone mass density; but buoyant and/or support activities such as swimming, rowing, and cycling—although excellent activities for developing cardiovascular health and fitness and maintaining body weight—do not have as much impact on bone health. Nevertheless, habitual physical activity, in itself, has the capacity to promote healthy bones and perhaps prevent the disabling outcomes from osteoporosis.

Low Back Pain

In general, the elderly are more likely to incur trauma to the lower back during activities associated with daily living than are younger individuals. There are several causes of low back pain in the elderly. Back pain usually occurs as a result of injury to the tissues surrounding the vertebral disk.[28] The extent of disability from low back pain can vary considerably. Assuredly, even minimal injury to the back can produce sufficient pain to restrict the desire to endure daily activities.

There is little indication that physical activity is related to the risk of back injury. However, habitual exercise can play an important role in the individual's response to back pain. When treatment for back disabilities includes physical activity, less depression occurs, which improves the person's attitude and self-esteem. Much of this improvement in attitude may result from gained mobility. Beneficial effects of motion exercises also suggest faster recovery from acute low back pain episodes.[29] However, exercise therapy for patients with low back pain varies according to the type of injury incurred. Acute back injuries should receive attention from the proper medical personnel. Undertaking activities should only begin after consulting with a physician. Most hospitals have outpatient back rehabilitation programs that can assist in rehabilitating acute injuries. Conversely, elderly individuals suffering from chronic low back pain may benefit from motion and muscle-strengthening exercises. Patients can improve their mobility through physical activity programs that incorporate motion exercises for the lower back. For many, the incorporation of these exercises provides hope for achieving self-reliance and the return to normal daily function.

Although physical activity does not in itself prevent low back pain, moderate exercise programs that encourage fitness and strength, can benefit individuals with chronic low back pain. The objective is to return these elderly patients to daily activities that promote independence and improve self-esteem.

Anxiety, Tension, and Mental Health

For the elderly, the aging process is frequently viewed with an anxious state of mind. Anxieties and tensions that result from fears of disability and death, often inhibit their ability to pursue daily activities. Resigned to a restricted lifestyle that decreases their functional status and encourages the deleterious effects of sedentary living, many elderly individuals jeopardize their quality of life. However, there is increasing evidence that exercise can improve mood states and affect overall mental health. Physical activity is an effective tool for improving mental health when it is defined as a positive mood state with infrequent feelings of anxiety and depression.[30] There are three areas in which habitual physical activity may impact mental health.[31] First, there is some evidence to suggest that physical activity prevents the onset of mental health problems. Second, habitual exercise may prevent mental health problems from escalating into situations that require medical attention or hospitalization. Finally, activity may prevent those with serious mental illnesses from needing advanced forms of medical attention.

Individuals who are active tend to be better satisfied with their lifestyle habits, which improves self-esteem and reduces depression.

Reasons for the positive influence of exercise on mood states is not fully understood. Physically active individuals are known to have higher levels of endorphin, a naturally released hormone with opium-like effects. High levels of this hormone are related to contented mood states.[32] In addition, poor sleeping habits can reduce alertness and increase depression, which alters the mental mood state. Physically active individuals improve their quality of sleep, which may rectify poor mood states. Finally, as discussed previously, exercise is an effective tool against obesity and other factors that favorably affect self-esteem. Improvements in mood state may be related to physical and behavioral self-observations in lifestyle habits. As exercise therapy progresses, individuals frequently report a greater overall satisfaction in health and well-being, which may translate to a better mood state. Elderly patients who lose weight are likely to feel better about themselves. Consequently, improving lifestyle habits through physical activity strengthens self-esteem and improves mental outlook. Mood states of the elderly individual may also be influenced by peer acceptance. Lost independence due to disabilities from aging can create feelings of withdrawal from social circles and from society as a whole. Preventing or delaying the loss of self-sufficiency by remaining physically active can encourage peer acceptance and increase social activity.

In general, increased participation in physical activity may provide the potential to improve and promote a healthy mental outlook. Elderly individuals who remain active are more likely to feel better about themselves and cope better under stressful conditions. Regardless of whether physical activity has an impact on physical, social, and/or behavioral mechanisms, one sure consequence of exercise is an improved mental state and, ultimately, an improved quality of life.

BEGINNING AN EXERCISE PROGRAM

Exercise Prescription for the Elderly

All the aging changes described thus far can only be said to accompany the aging process. We can infer that changes in these various functional capacities observed in different groups of subjects at increasing age levels may result from a combination of at least three factors:

1. true aging phenomena,

2. unrecognized disease processes whose incidence and severity increase with age,

3. disuse phenomena or the increasing sedentariness of our lifestyle as we grow older.

Since we can do little to modify the first two factors, and since the third factor offers the potential for being modified by the methods of conditioning and training already known to the health and physical education professions, we must now focus our attention to how trainable, from an exercise perspective, is the older human body.

Physical Training in the Older Adult

The trainability of elderly men and women alike and the effectiveness of physical activity have been demonstrated through research. Older adults who become more physically active gain in cardiovascular endurance, strength and muscular endurance, and in flexibility. How much they improve depends on their initial level of fitness and the types of activities they select as part of their training program (i.e., walking, jogging, strength training, etc.).

In regard to strength development, the elderly can expect to increase their strength levels, but the amount of muscle enlargement or hypertrophy one can expect to achieve generally decreases with age. In relation to body composition, after age sixty, inactive adults continue to gain body fat while decreasing lean body weight despite the tendency toward lower body weight.[33]

Although hypokinesis (deterioration) results in the declining functional capacity of the body's physical capacity at any age, the rate of decline is accelerated in the over-twenty-five age group. It is critical therefore, that the aging individual understands the urgency of becoming or remaining active or both. It must also be emphasized that age is no barrier to exercise and that the aging body will respond to physical training in much the same way as the young body. The only real difference is that the time frame (weeks or months) required for the training response will usually be longer for older persons, and the ultimate level of fitness that one can hope to achieve will likely be lower as age progresses.

The guidelines used to prescribe exercise for young and older populations are generally not different. It does become necessary, however, to alter intensity levels and to look at some special considerations for exercise with regard to the inevitable aging process.

Generally, exercise is considered a safe activity for most individuals. Older adults who wish to take part in an exercise program should have a complete medical exam, including a stress electrocardiogram as recommended by the American College of Sports Medicine (ACSM). This type of test should be administered to:

1. men over age forty and women over age fifty;

2. persons with a total cholesterol level above 200 mg/dl, or an HDL-cholesterol below 35 mg/dl;

3. hypertensive and diabetic patients;

4. cigarette smokers;

5. individuals with a family history of CHD (coronary heart disease), syncope (fainting), or sudden death before age sixty;

6. people with an abnormal resting electrocardiogram;

7. all individuals with symptoms of chest discomfort, dysrhythmias, syncope, or chronic incompetence (a heart rate that increases slowly during exercise and never reaches maximum).[34]

Developing Muscular Strength and Endurance

It is our belief that limitations on exercise in the adult years and beyond are usually self-imposed by a lack of consistency and continuity in an individual's exercise habits. Almost every activity that is mastered during one's childhood can be continued by a healthy individual well into old age. This is true, however, only if participation occurs a minimum of three times per week. If professional and/or social obligations prevent this degree of participation, calisthenics or weight training programs can be accomplished during the week in order to prevent the weekend activity from becoming too much of a strain. Suitable calisthenic or weight training exercises from a trained physical educator can help the elderly maintain muscular strength and flexibility, while the application of swimming, walking and/or jogging programs can maintain cardiorespiratory fitness.

In order to make exercise activities more enjoyable, challenging, and self-motivating, it is most important that every healthy individual be skilled in one or several sport activities that are vigorous enough to maintain optimum cardiorespiratory fitness. Activities that are considered drudgery are not likely to be continued for long no matter what benefits may be derived. Excellent activities that meet the above criteria are swimming, walking, jogging (as mentioned earlier), tennis, handball, racquet ball, volleyball, cycling, badminton, and skiing.

One caution before you begin a program of weight training. Because blood circulation tends to be impeded during weight training (especially with isometrics), you should not undertake such a program without close medical supervision if you have a history of coronary heart disease, circulatory problems, or hypertension (high blood pressure). However, increased strength can benefit individuals with hypertension because the blood pressure response to a muscle load is less in people who are stronger.

Getting Started

Self-initiating physical activity is important for all individuals if they want to prevent the deleterious effects of a sedentary lifestyle. However, since the elderly population is quite diverse with regard to its functional abilities and health limitations, greater emphasis must be placed on obtaining appropriate medical screening and supervision. Knowing where to turn to begin an exercise program can alleviate a lot of anxieties. Participants need to understand what activities are appropriate or how much physical activity is necessary. Trained health professionals are available to educate and orient the elderly and caregivers to physical activity programming. Most professionals can be contacted through hospital or community-based exercise programs. When investigating a program or the attending health professional, be sure both have the appropriate license. Any exercise program should be run by a certified fitness professional. The American College of Sports Medicine certifies exercise specialists who are trained in both preventive and rehabilitative exercise therapy. These professionals should have current CPR and first aid certifications. In addition, be sure that the fitness program or professional has a medical emergency plan of action. Finally, if necessary, be sure that exercise programming can accommodate any pertinent disabilities. With this in mind, exploring the options for exercise programs can begin.

Most communities have exercise programming managed by local senior citizen centers or school-related staffs. These programs are often designed specifically with elderly individuals in mind. An added benefit to community-based programs includes the chance to develop a social support network with individuals of similar age and circumstance. Often these exercise programs provide additional events for opportunities to socialize. Additionally, physical activity programming may be found in hospital-supported programs. Hospitals that conduct outpatient cardiac rehabilitation programs often extend exercise services to individuals within the community. Once again, these programs provide opportunities for group exercise in a social setting. Trained medical personnel are staffed to conduct exercise in these facilities for both healthy and diseased populations. Another option is to employ a certified exercise specialist for personal instruction. Most certified trainers work out of a fitness facility but many will assist and supervise programs in the individual's home. Home exercise can provide a more relaxed atmosphere in comfortable surroundings. This can be advantageous for individuals who are extremely uncomfortable exercising in public or lack the flexibility in their schedule to fit into group classes. However, several disadvantages to home exercise exist. Frequently, the home exercise participant is compelled to purchase expensive exercise equipment for indoor use. Moreover, home programs eliminate the social aspects of group exercise unless a workout partner is included.

One added disadvantage to using a health professional either at home or in hospital-based programs can be the expense. Health coverage for exercise instruction may vary according to insurance programs and should be investigated prior to beginning a supervised exercise program. Community programs are usually more affordable and in many cases are free to senior citizens within the community.

While supervised exercise instruction is strongly recommended, it may be unattainable for certain elderly individuals. This should not excuse anyone from becoming more physically active, however. Clearly, older adults who wish to begin a program of physical activity should first consult with their physician. Inquiries should be made concerning which activities are appropriate and what physical limitations need clarified to the elderly persons. Oftentimes a daily walking program for 30 to 60 minutes is both possible and safe for most individuals and can protect against the hazards of sedentary living. Additionally, physicians are usually able to direct patients to exercise therapy programs that are most appropriate given their specific circumstances.

Another consideration to beginning physical activity programming for the elderly is exercise adherence. In general, keeping to an exercise program is difficult for elderly people. This may be due to the misconception that many elderly have about their activity levels: they perceive themselves as more physically active than they really are. This misunderstanding can lead older people to put off initiating exercise programs. Furthermore, those who do begin such programs often battle their inconsistency in keeping up with a daily exercise routine. To combat the problem of exercise adherence many researchers suggest exercising with a partner or group. In fact, this is one advantage to group exercise programs: those who exercise in this manner are more likely to persevere. In addition, keeping an exercise diary that tracks the duration or distance of each exercise session can allow exercisers to record their accomplishments. Moreover, short-term goals can be added to the diary. For instance, efforts at small amounts of weight loss, the ability to get out of a chair unaided, the ability to walk a given distance, and many others. As improvements are made and goals are met, exercisers can evaluate their progression. The use of a physical activity diary assists in motivating participants by providing sound evidence of their achievements. Finally, another motivational aid is positive reinforcement. Complimenting the improvements that are made encourages participants to continue exercising.

Several alternatives exist for physical activity programming. Determining which is appropriate may depend on the accessability and expense involved. Nevertheless, special attention to the specific needs and health limitations of the elderly must be considered when implementing a physical activity program. Whether through a health professional or a physician, individuals should be oriented and encouraged to maintain a physically active lifestyle that encourages self-sufficiency and improves their quality of life.

Activity Guidelines for the Elderly

1. Be sure to consult a physician before beginning an exercise program.

2. Always begin your exercise program with a 10- to 15-minute warm-up. This time is needed to prepare the body for exertion. Begin with stretching exercises to loosen up muscles, then move on to light exercise such as mild walking or stationary bicycling. Be sure to stretch all the major muscle groups with emphasis on the muscles that will be utilized for the particular exercises you will be doing.

3. Start easy. Ten minutes of light-to-moderate exercise is a good start for your first session. As your exercise tolerance improves, try adding 5 more minutes every couple of weeks. Slowly work up to 30 to 60 minutes of light-to-moderate exercise.

4. The exercise intensity should not cause you to break a sweat. If you become overheated, ease up! If the activity feels too hard, then slow down. You will benefit more by extending the duration of the activity than by working harder.

5. When finishing an exercise, don't stop right away. Rather, begin to slow the pace down. Maintain this easy pace for 5 to 10 minutes.

6. Try incorporating more activity into your daily schedule. If you drive a car for short distances, try walking. If you always seek the closest parking spot to the door, try parking further back and walking. Take the stairs not the elevator.

7. If you're a shut in, try walking around one floor of your home 2 to 3 times a day. With the permission of your physician, include some stair-climbing a couple times.

8. Practice sitting and standing from a hard back but sturdy chair; this will help to strengthen the legs.

9. Find a partner to exercise with at home if you are unable to attend a group exercise program.

10. Finally, know the signs of overexertion. If you feel chest pain, shortness of breath, nausea, or numbness, stop exercising and consult your physician.

A CONTINUING HOME EXERCISE PROGRAM FOR THE ELDERLY

The following list of home exercises are provided for the home-care provider and the elderly to assist in the development of a personal health and fitness program for older adults. All of the following exercises can be done without the use of specialized equipment. Please note that the number of repetitions and sets (or groups of repetitions) should be determined by the readiness level of the elder and the stress caused by the exercise. Certain individuals with physical limitations should proceed with caution if signs or symptoms of intolerance to specific exercises occur. *Always consult your physician before starting any excercise program.*

1. *Side Straddle Hops*

   Purpose: Accelerate heart rate and stretch major muscle groups.

   Starting Position: Feet together with arms at sides.

   Count 1: Swing arms over head and spread feet apart.

   Count 2: Return to starting position.

2. *Thighs-Toes-Thighs-Up*

   Purpose: Stretch hamstrings (the back of the legs).

   Starting Position: Feet together with arms extended over head.

   Count 1: Bring arms forward and touch knees with hands.

   Count 2: Continue flexing forward at the hips to touch the toes.

   Count 3: Begin extension at the hips to touch knees.

   Count 4: Return to starting position.

3. *Four-Count Toe Touch*

   Purpose: Stretch inner thigh muscles, hamstrings, and the sides of the abdomen.

   Starting Position: Arms extended straight forward with thumbs interlocked and feet wide apart.

   Count 1: Flex at hips and touch fingers to left foot.

   Count 2: Touch floor between feet with the hands.

   Count 3: Touch fingers to right foot.

   Count 4: Return to starting position.

4. *Front Leg Stretch*

   Purpose: Stretch muscles in the backs of thighs.

   Starting Position: Prone (lying on chest) with right knee flexed and right hand around right ankle.

   Count 1: Slowly pull ankle to hip and hold three to five seconds.

   Count 2: Return leg to floor.

5. *Knee Pushups*

   Purpose: Strengthen muscles of the arms and chest.

   Starting Position: Chest on floor with one hand on either side of the chest, palm down. Legs are extended to the rear.

   Count 1: Push body up while extending elbows while your knees remain on the floor.

   Count 2: Return to starting position.

6. *Trunk Rotation*

   Purpose: Stretch muscles in the shoulder girdle and sides of the trunk.

   Starting Position: Arms extended to the side at shoulder level with feet wide apart.

   Count 1: Twist trunk to the left and continue with arms as far as possible.

   Count 2: Return to starting position.

   Count 3: Twist trunk to the right and continue with arms as far as possible.

   Count 4: Return to starting position.

7. *Heel Raises*

   Purpose: Stretch and strengthen calf muscles.

   Starting Position: Feet approximately shoulder-width apart with arms positioned for balance.

   Count 1: Raise heels off the floor to maximum point.

   Count 2: Return to starting position.

   (Note: A board can be placed under the toes to increase the range of motion.)

8. *Small Arm Circles*

   Purpose: Stretch and strengthen shoulder muscles.

   Starting Position: Arms extended to the side at shoulder level with feet positioned for balance.

   Count 1: Rotate shoulders so that arms make small forward circles in succession.

   Count 2: Reverse the direction of the arms so that they make small backward circles in succession.

9. *Leg Adductions*

   Purpose: Stretch and strengthen leg and side abdominal muscles.

   Starting Position: Resting on side, top leg raised in the air approximately 18 inches (or whatever height less than this that can be managed), and hand of top arm placed on floor in front of the chest for leverage.

   Count 1: While keeping top leg in the air, raise bottom leg until it touches the inner part of top leg.

   Count 2: Return to starting position.

   (Note: Repeat through selected number of repetitions and then switch sides to exercise the other side of the body.)

10. *Double Leg Raising and Lowering*

    Purpose: Stretch and strengthen leg and abdominal muscles.

    Starting position: Lying on your back with legs outstretched.

    Count 1: Elevate both legs to an eighty or ninety degree angle (or whatever height less than this that can be managed) with the floor, keeping the knees straight.

    Count 2: Return to starting position.

Elders who are bed-ridden also need motion exercises. They can practice the following exercises 5 to 15 repetitions, 2 to 3 times a day. As the individual improves, the exercises can be done sitting up. Finally, progress to standing while doing the exercises.

Slow, deep breathing.

Shoulder shrugs

Arm circles

Ankle flexion and extensions

Knee to chest

CASE STUDIES

The following are case studies of elderly individuals who started fitness programs late in life and now, through appropriate training and guidance, are self-sufficient in their exercise programs as well as much healthier and happier.

Case 1

A seventy-three-year-old retired college physics professor from the University of Maryland was seen for a routine medical screening evaluation. His father had experienced a heart attack at age sixty-two years, as did a half-brother at age sixty-nine years. Twenty-one percent of his total body weight was fat, indicating the need to lose 20 pounds of fat. He was advised of having five coronary heart disease risk factors (excess fat, very low endurance capacity, elevated serum cholesterol, high blood pressure, and a family history of coronary heart disease).

He was placed on a low-fat, low-calorie diet and a home walking program, working up to four miles per day over a six-week period. A friend was instructed in blood pressure recording, and a diary was kept. When retested three months later, he had lost fourteen pounds of fat weight and his endurance capacity from walking every day had improved dramatically. The serum cholesterol as well as blood pressure also decreased considerably during this period.

Case 2

A seventy-five-year-old former businessman was evaluated because of frequently occurring minor chest pain. The medical history was significant in that his father died at age sixty-one years of a heart attack. Twenty-three percent of his total body weight was fat, which contributed significantly to his excess weight. He also was found to have very high blood pressure (190/120) and elevated total cholesterol (338 mg/dl). Although his resting electrocardiogram was normal, an exercise electrocardiogram indicated multiple coronary risk factors. Six weeks later, while on a golfing vacation, he experienced several episodes of chest pain. An electrocardiogram taken the following day revealed that he had suffered a mild heart attack. After a two-week hospital stay, he was discharged and began a home walking and exercise regimen. Two months later, he underwent another medical evaluation before entering a hospital-based exercise program. On evaluation, it was found that percent body fat (and total body weight), cholesterol, and blood pressure had all decreased favorably and that another exercise electrocardiogram performed on him had also improved. He began at a low level of exercise in the hospital-based exercise program and has progressed to brisk walking and slow jogging activities with no adverse physical problems or difficulties.

NOTES

1. H. H. Jones, J. D. Priest, W. C. Hayes, C. Tichenor, and D. A. Nagle, "Humeral Hypertrophy in Response to Exercise," *Journal of Bone and Joint Surgery* 59A (1977): 204.

2. Ibid.

3. M. B. Fischer and J. E. Birren, "Age and Strength," *Journal of Psychology* 31 (1947): 490.

4. K. Rodahl, "Physical Work Capacity," *Archives of Environmental Health* 2 (1961): 499.

5. Fischer and Birren, "Age and Strength," and Rodahl, "Physical Work Capacity."

6. S. Makrides, "Protein Synthesis and Degradation During Aging and Senescence," *Biological Review* 58 (1983): 343.

7. E. Smith and R. Serfass (eds.), *Exercise and Aging* (Hillside, N.J., Enslow Publishers, 1981).

8. Ibid.

9. H. A. deVries, R. A. Wiswell, G. T. Romero, and E. Heckathome, "Changes with Age in Monosynaptic Reflexes Elicited by Mechanical and Electrical Stimulation," *American Journal of Physiological Medicine* 64 (1985): 71.

10. Ibid.

11. J. E. Birren, H. A. Imus, and W. F. Windle (eds.), *The Process of Aging in the Nervous System* (Springfield, Ill.: Charles C. Thomas, 1959).

12. P. M. Clarkson, "The Effect of Age and Activity Level on Fractionated Response Time," *Medicine and Science in Sports and Exercise* 10 (1978): 66; deVries et al., "Changes with Age in Monosynaptic Reflexes Elicited by Mechanical

and Electrical Stimulation"; D. E. Sherwood and D. J. Selder, "Cardiorespiratory Health, Reaction Time, and Aging," *Medicine and Science in Sports and Exercise* 11 (1979): 186; W. W. Spirduso, "Exercise and the Aging Brain," *Research Quarterly for Exercise and Sport* 54 (1953): 208; and W. W. Spirduso and R. R. Farrar, "Effects of Aerobic Training on Reactive Capacity: An Animal Model," *Journal of Gerontology* 36 (1981): 654.

13. Spirduso and Farrar, "Effects of Aerobic Training on Reactive Capacity: An Animal Model."

14. Ibid.

15. G. Bray, *The Obese Patient* (Philadelphia: W. B. Saunders, 1976), and R. Shephard, *Physical Activity and Aging* (Chicago: Year Book Medical Publishers, 1978).

16. Bray, *The Obese Patient.*

17. Ibid.

18. Ibid.

19. Ibid.

20. Sherwood and Selder, "Cardiorespiratory Health, Reaction Time, and Aging," *Medicine and Science in Sports and Exercise* 11 (1979): 186.

21. C. Bouchard, R. Shephard, T. Stevens, J. Sutton, and B. McPherson, *Exercise, Fitness and Health* (Champaign, Ill.: Human Kinetics, 1990).

22. R. Rauramaa, J. Salonen, K. Seppanen, R. Salonen, J. Venalainen, M. Ihanainen, and V. Rissanen, "Inhibition of Plattlet Aggregability by Moderate Intensity Exercise: A Randomized Clinical Trial in Overweight Men," *Circulation* 74 (1986): 939–44.

23. Bouchard et al., *Exercise, Fitness and Health.*

24. P. Lee, and C. Estes, *The Nation's Health* (Boston: Jones and Bartlett Co., 1990).

25. Bouchard et al., *Exercise, Fitness and Health.*

26. Ibid.

27. H. J. Montoye, E. L. Smith, D. F. Fardon, and E. T. Howley, "Bone Mineral in Senior Tennis Players," *Scandinavian Journal of Sports Science* 2 (1980): 26.

28. Bouchard et al., *Exercise, Fitness and Health.*

29. M. Bergquist-Ullman, and U. Larsson, "Acute Low Back Pain in Industry: A Controlled Prospective Study with Special Reference to Therapy and Confounding Factors," *Acta Orthop Scand* 170 (1977): 1–117.

30. Bouchard et al., *Exercise, Fitness and Health.*

31. G. Caplan, *Principles of Preventive Psychiatry* (New York: Basic Books, 1954).

32. Bouchard et al., *Exercise, Fitness and Health.*

33. Bray, *The Obese Patient.*

34. American College of Sports Medicine, *Guidelines for Graded Exercise Testing and Prescription* (Philadelphia: Lea and Febiger, 1992).

ADDITIONAL REFERENCES

American Heart Association, Lipid Disorders Conference, Washington University, St. Louis, Mo., 1990.

Edington, D. W.; A. C. Cosmas, and W. B. McCafferty. "Exercise and Longevity: Evidence for a Threshold Age," *Journal of Gerontology* 27 (1972): 341.

Moritani, T., and H. A. deVries. "Neural Factors Versus Hypertrophy in the Time Course of Muscle Strength Gain in Young and Old Men. *Journal of Gerontology* 36 (1981): 294.

Stephens, T. "Physical Activity and Mental Health in the United States and Canada: Evidence from Four Population Studies," *Preventive Medicine* 17 (1988): 35–47.

9

Quackery and the Elderly

Dawn Larsen, Ph.D.

Each year American consumers spend roughly $10 billion on medical quackery—remedies and devices that are scientifically unproven. These devices are ineffective, often expensive, and sometimes harmful. There are also tremendous indirect costs of health quackery resulting from a delay in legitimate treatment or from injury by a "quack" treatment.

People who sell unproven treatments are called quacks. They have been around since the days of the traveling "snake oil" salesman who claimed that his products cured nearly everything. However, the methods of today's quacks have changed. Their products are now sold through advertisements, phony sales corporations, foundations, and clinics.

Though people of all ages can be fooled by quackery, the largest group of victims is among the older population. The impact of fraud on the elderly is so severe that a four-year investigation on quackery was conducted by the Subcommittee on Health and Long-Term Care, of the U.S. House of Representatives. Results of the study were published in a report titled "Quackery: A $10 Billion Scandal." Its conclusions indicated that 60 percent of all victims of healthcare fraud were older persons.

Older people tend to have more long-term, chronic illnesses and disabilities compared to younger people. These conditions include arthritis, diabetes, and cancer. This makes older people more vulnerable to quacks, who will offer hope and relief to unhappy, often desperate people. Victims often resort to quackery because of fear, loss of hope, and poor or inadequate information. The National Institute on Aging has noted that three of the primary targets for health quackery among the elderly are arthritis, cancer, and the aging process itself.[1] Each of these areas deserves special emphasis.

ARTHRITIS

Arthritis is a chronic disease that causes aches, pains, or swelling in joints, muscles, and fibrous tissues. The major types of arthritis often have periods of remission, when symptoms recede or disappear. Individuals may be free of pain or discomfort for days, weeks, or even months. This makes it difficult even for medical professionals to judge the effectiveness of some treatments. If this remission follows the use of an unorthodox or quack remedy, people often mistakenly associate the remedy with relief. In one year alone, the Arthritis Foundation estimated that for every dollar spent on arthritis research, $25 was spent on arthritis quackery.[2]

A study by the Food and Drug Administration has summarized why arthritis sufferers are especially vulnerable to quackery:

1. Arthritis is usually a chronic ailment for which there is no cure.

2. Many do not know how to get the best possible help for arthritis. When they seek medical help, treatment by unqualified physicians is often unsatisfactory.

3. Arthritis often causes great discomfort. Sufferers fear their condition might get worse and impair their ability to function.

4. Frustration and disappointment may cause people to lose faith in orthodox treatment, and so they grasp at "miracle" treatments.[3]

There are many types of unorthodox treatment methods. These include mechanical devices, dietary supplements, fad diets, environmental methods, and acupuncture, as well as some medications. Some of these methods may seriously impair health and could even be fatal. Others may not directly cause harm, but may keep people from seeking treatment from qualified physicians.

Probably the best-known mechanical device for alleviating arthritis pain is the copper bracelet. Modern folklore suggests that copper bracelets worn on both wrists can set up "curative circuits."[4] However, there is no evidence to support this theory. Other devices include vibrators and whirlpools, which may carry exaggerated claims that they relieve arthritis. While vibrators may relieve some muscle tension, they sometimes increase joint inflammation. In many cases whirlpool baths are no more effective than simple hot baths. These devices should not be purchased without first consulting a physician. Other devices claiming to cure arthritis, such as vibrating mattresses, brass tubes with supposed healing powers, and solar mattress boards, have been removed from the market by the FDA.

There have also been claims that certain types of environments can cure or relieve arthritis symptoms. In 1974, a mining company in Boulder, Colorado, claimed that radon gas from an abandoned uranium mine could relieve arthritis.[5] The radon level in the mine was actually too low to have any type of effect. This was fortunate, since high levels of radon have been associated with an increased risk of developing cancer. Warm climates have sometimes been promoted as areas where arthritis sufferers will feel better. Weather does not alter the course of arthritis, and the "weather myth" may have arisen because some people feel better when the barometric pressure drops.[6]

Though the Arthritis Foundation states that no specific food, diet, or supplement can help arthritis, a number of products have been promoted for this purpose. These products include cod liver oil, bee and snake venom, "immune milk," and Oxycal (a vitamin C supplement with calcium). Green-lipped mussel was marketed under a number of product names that claimed to be effective against arthritis.

Many people have been taken in by claims of arthritis relief at unethical clinics in the United States and nearby countries. These clinics may offer a combination of physical therapy and medication. Physical therapy may feature mineral waters where temporary relief can be due to simple rest and relaxation. Other procedures can involve special diets, enemas, massage, and the use of potentially dangerous drugs such as steroids. Clinics in Canada, Mexico, and the Dominican Republic, as well as the United States, have offered expensive treatments not based on sound research or established medical practice.[7]

According to the Arthritis Foundation, people should suspect unproven remedies if they:

1. claim to work for all types of arthritis;

2. use only case histories or testimonials as proof;

3. use only one study as proof;

4. use a study without a control group;

5. do not list contents;

6. have no warnings about side effects;

7. are described as harmless or natural;

8. claim to be based on a secret formula;

9. are available from only one source;

10. or are promoted only through the media, books, or mail order.[8]

People suffering from arthritis, and those who care for them, can obtain reliable information about appropriate treatment from the Arthritis Foundation or one of its local offices. These offices should be listed in your local phone directory.

The following books contain reliable and helpful information:

Arthritis: A Comprehensive Guide to Understanding Your Arthritis, James F. Fries, M.S., Addison-Wesley Publishing Company, Reading, Mass., 1986.

The Arthritis Helpbook: A Tested Self-Management Program for Coping with Your Arthritis, Kate Lorig, R.N., Dr.P.H., Addison-Wesley Publishing Company, Reading, Mass., 1986.

Understanding Arthritis: What It Is, How It's Treated, How to Cope With It, the Arthritis Foundation Staff, Charles Scribner's Sons, New York, 1985.[9]

The Arthritis Foundation has specific criteria for medical accuracy and scientific validity. The following books do not meet these criteria:

Arthritis Can Be Cured—A Layman's Guide, by Bernard Aschner, M.D.

Arthritis, Nutrition and Natural Therapy, by Calson Wade.

The Arthritic's Cookbook, by Colin M. Dong, M.D., and Jane Banks.

A Doctor's Proven New Home Cure for Arthritis, by Giraud W. Campbell, D.O., and R. Stone.

Bees Don't Get Arthritis, by Fred Malone.

The Miraculous Holistic Balanced Treatment for Arthritic Diseases, by Henry B. Rothblaft, J.D., L.L.M., Donna Pinorsky, R.N., and Michael Brodsky.

The Nightshades and Health, by Normal Franklin Childers and Gerard M. Russo.

Pain-Free Arthritis, by Dvera Berson with Sander Roy.

There Is a Cure for Arthritis, by Paavo O. Airola, N.D.

You Can Stay Well and *Let's Get Well,* both by Adele Davis, M.S.[10]

Certain guidelines have been developed for arthritis sufferers and those who love and care for them. These guidelines are intended to help foster intelligent and informed decision making.

1. Leave the diagnosis of ailments to the physician.

2. Let the physician prescribe the medications.

3. Be cautious about testimonials. Some may be lies, and some results may be due to the spontaneous remission of the disease.

4. Be careful of those who promise a "sure cure" or claim to have a secret formula for arthritis.

5. Avoid products claiming to offer more than temporary relief from the minor pain of arthritis, unless your physician prescribes them.

6. Check with your physician before using over-the-counter medications that make specific claims to relieve symptoms.

7. Be aware that there is no specific cure for arthritis.

8. Avoid spas or clinics that encourage self-diagnosis or claim that treatments like mineral baths have therapeutic value.

9. Be aware that product claims are not necessarily true just because the product is marketed.

10. Contact a local Arthritis Foundation chapter for assistance.[11]

CANCER

Cancer is currently the second leading cause of death in the United States, accounting for one-fifth of all deaths. Like arthritis, cancer occurs more often in older people. They are consequently more vulnerable to quacks, who exploit the older person's fear of cancer by offering cures or treatments with no documented value.

Simply stated, cancer is the general term for malignant tumors. This term may refer to a large number of diseases caused by abnormal cell growth. Because the cells are abnormal, they have no useful function and can actually harm or destroy other body cells. Treatment can be complicated and long because "bad" cells must be destroyed with minimal damage to normal cells. Though specific causes are unknown, a number of risk factors have been identified. These risk factors, in turn, interact with individual heredity and the environment.

There are several types of orthodox cancer treatments that may be used together to increase effectiveness. These include surgery, radiation therapy, and chemotherapy. However, there are many types of costly quack treatments that focus on fears that cancers are incurable. These fears may be especially sharp among older people who dread infirmity and have a limited income.

One reason unorthodox therapy may be appealing is that its methods are explained in simple terms that seem believable to patients, especially those who are emotionally vulnerable and desperate. Some common (but false) explanations are:

1. Cancer is a symptom, not a disease.

2. Symptoms are caused by diet, stress, or environment.

3. Fitness, nutrition, and mental attitude allow for physical and mental defense against cancer.

4. Conventional medical therapy treats the symptoms, not the disease—and "weakens" the body's reserves.[12]

People may fall prey to cancer quackery regardless of their educational background or income level. Nontraditional or unorthodox treatments may seem effective for several reasons:

1. Some patients who believe they have been cured of cancer may never have had it in the first place.

2. Those who use unproven methods as well as conventional treatments may mistakenly believe improvement resulted from the unproven methods.

3. Most cancer patients feel better on some days than others. If a period of apparent relief follows an unproven treatment, patients may think they're "improved" or "cured."

4. Doctors may be very cautious or conservative in communicating with patients. Some patients may try quack cures and live longer than predicted by a doctor. They may then think the quack remedy was effective, when in fact the doctor's prediction was too pessimistic.[13]

Cancer quackery may be as old as the first recorded case of this disease. Reports from the American Cancer Society indicate that over seventy types of unorthodox remedies have appeared in just the last fifty years. Like arthritis remedies, they are ineffective and sometimes harmful.

One of the most unsavory "folk remedies" was ADS, which was marketed as an herbal tea. It was sold by a California physician, Bruce Halstead, who charged as much as $150 per quart. The "tea" was analyzed and found to by 99.4 percent water. The rest was a thick paste containing bacteria found in human waste. Halstead was convicted of cancer fraud and grand theft in 1986. Called "a crook selling swamp water" by the prosecuting attorney, he was fined $10,000 and sentenced to four years in jail.[14]

Other approaches have focused on meditation and counseling. O. Carl Simonton, a physician from Texas, suggests the brain can secrete a substance to help the immune system attack cancer cells. He noted that some cancer patients with "positive attitudes" seemed to recover faster and live longer than those who were not as optimistic. This observation led to the development of a system for motivating "positive attitudes." One exercise encourages patients to imagine their cancer cells being destroyed by their own immune systems. This strategy was used by the late Gilda Radner in her battle against ovarian cancer.[15] Though Simonton's theory is physically harmless, it may keep patients from using more conventional therapy. The American Cancer Society has not endorsed this procedure, and has questioned studies supporting this treatment.[16]

Ineffective and unproven diagnostic tests have also been part of quack cancer treatments. Two such tests were developed by dentist William Kelley, whose patients included the late actor Steve McQueen. One test was based on the idea that cancer was a foreign protein. Kelley suggested that cancer was caused by eating the wrong kinds of protein. Kelley claimed that the other test, the Kelley Malignancy Test, could show the presence, growth rate, age, and location of tumors, as well as determine treatment and regulate medicine.[17]

The American Dental Association reported that Kelley was convicted in 1970 of practicing medicine without a license. According to witnesses, he had diagnosed lung cancer by examining blood from a patient's finger. He had also prescribed supplements and a special diet as a form of treatment.[18] His license to practice dentistry was later suspended on the basis of complaints that he had offered cancer diagnosis and treatment in his dental office. Even after the suspension, Kelley continued treating patients through an organization called the International Health Institute.[19]

Several unproven cancer remedies have received national news coverage. One is Immuno-Augmentative Therapy (IAT), based on the idea that cancer can be treated by activating an immune defense system. Its proponent was zoologist Lawrence Burton. He established an expensive clinic in the Bahamas after his request to test humans in the United States was denied by the Food and Drug Administration. Burton also provided guidelines recommending that patients consult attorneys about forcing insurance companies to pay for IAT.[20]

Although IAT was given favorable publicity by the news program "60 Minutes," a featured patient whose "miraculous recovery" was attributed to IAT died two weeks after the broadcast. Viewers were not informed of this, and the public was left with a positive impression of IAT. Two states, Florida and Oklahoma, enacted laws permitting the use of IAT in 1981. Florida, however, repealed its law two years later.

An in-depth investigation of IAT was begun after treatment products were analyzed in 1985. The products were obtained from patients and tested in the state of Washington. This analysis indicated that the products were contaminated with Hepatitis B and HIV viruses. The samples were then referred to the United States Centers for Disease Control in Atlanta, where live HIV virus was discovered in one of the samples.[21]

Laetrile has been one of the most controversial unproven remedies. It is the trade name for amygdalin, which is found in the kernels, or pits, of apricots and several other plants. It contains several substances, like the sugar glucose, which are harmless. However, it also contains cyanide, which is a poison.

Several theories have been offered in support of laetrile as a cancer therapy. However, other evidence indicates that laetrile can damage healthy cells. Thirty-seven cases of poisoning and 17 deaths from laetrile and laetrile-containing fruit kernels have been described by Dr. Joseph F. Ross, professor of medicine and pathology at UCLA School of Medicine.[22] Dr. Victor Herbert believes that cyanide in laetrile may actually have caused or accelerated some deaths that were attributed to cancer.[23]

Though laetrile is no longer promoted as a cancer cure, supporters claim that it prevents or stops cancer growth, alleviates pain, and promotes well-being. Treatment frequently includes coffee enemas, vitamin supplements, and a diet with little or no red meat. This treatment may be referred to as "holistic" or "metabolic" therapy.

The laetrile controversy prompted a clinical study by the Mayo Clinic and three other U.S. cancer centers in 1982. Sponsored by the National Cancer institute, the study focused on 178 terminal cancer patients. These patients received laetrile and the "metabolic therapy" recommended by laetrile advocates. Results did not in any way support the use of laetrile. No patients were cured and none experienced any relief from cancer symptoms. Tumor size actually increased in those who survived seven months. In addition, several had symptoms of cyanide poisoning or dangerous levels of cyanide in their blood.[24]

Though there have been several legal disputes over the availability of laetrile, the Food and Drug Administration has not approved its use for any illness. In addition, laetrile cannot be legally manufactured or carried between states in the United States. Discussing the controversial drug in 1977, *Consumer Reports* stated, "In our opinion, the use of laetrile as a treatment for the terminally ill cancer patient stands in violation of basic patient rights against being duped and offered a false sense of hope."[25]

Another compound once proposed as a cancer treatment was krebiozen. This is a powder containing an amino acid found in meat. Its use was advocated by Dr. Andrew C. Ivy, a respected scientist, researcher, and university official. However, five hundred of Dr. Ivy's krebiozen-treated cancer cases were reviewed by six prominent physicians, who found no evidence that cancer had been cured, reduced, or arrested, or that krebiozen could prolong life.[26]

The American Cancer Society has identified several ways in which people learn about, and are duped by unproven cancer treatments.

1. People may have friends or acquaintances who claim to have been cured or improved by a quack treatment.

2. Books promoting unproven cancer treatments are cleverly marketed and sell well. Some examples include:

   Happy People Rarely Get Cancer, by J. I. Rodale, 1972.

   The Incredible Story of Krebiozen: A Matter of Life or Death, by Herbert Bailey, 1962.

Laetrile Case Histories, by John A. Richardson, M.D., 1977.

Laetrile: Control for Cancer, by Glen D. Kittles, 1963.

Vitamin B-17: Forbidden Weapon Against Cancer, by Michael Culbert, 1974.

World Without Cancer, by G. Edward Griffen, 1974.

Skillfully written and well-marketed books like these may be dangerously convincing to those who don't question their information and principles.

3. Organizations that promote unproven methods of cancer treatment. These include: the Cancer Control Society, People Against Cancer, The National Health Federation, The Foundaton for Alternatives in Cancer Therapy Inc., and the International Association of Cancer Victors and Friends. Each group is well organized, subsidizing publications and conventions to attract followers.

4. Radio and television shows featuring advocates or promoters of unproven cancer treatments.

5. Testimonials, endorsements, or sponsorship by celebrities, entertainers, athletes, or socially prominent people.

There are a number of sources for reliable information on cancer treatment. One of the most convenient may be the local chapter of the American Cancer Society listed in your telephone book. The Cancer Information Service (CIS) may be contacted by calling 1-800-4-CANCER. Callers will be connected to the CIS offices in a specific area. Exceptions to this number are Washington, D.C., (1-202-636-5700), Alaska (1-800-638-6070), and Hawaii (1-800-524-6070). Physicians can refer to a database on treatments and results maintained by the National Cancer Institute.

Reliable books about cancer, written for consumers, include:

All About Cancer, Jay S. Roth, Philadelphia. The George F. Stickley Co., 1985.

The American Cancer Society's Complete Book of Cancer: Prevention, Detection, Treatment, Rehabilitation, Cure, Arthur Holleb, M.D. (ed.), New York, Doubleday & Co., 1986.

Guidelines for cancer patients have been offered by Wallace Janssen in a publication for the Food and Drug Administration:

1. Do not risk life or health on techniques that have not been approved.

2. Seek the best possible treatment offered by recognized experts.

3. Stay away from "fad" treatments advocated by people with no medical or scientific background.

4. Don't trust testimonials or people claiming to have been cured or improved by unrecognized treatments.

5. Continue with a prescribed treatment even if you do not see results right away.

6. Place trust in qualified health professionals whose careers involve cancer research and treatment.

7. If a specialist "gives up," choose another doctor. Good physicians do not abandon patients and leave them with no hope.[27]

ANTI-AGING PRODUCTS

Americans seem obsessed with a youthful appearance and specific standards of beauty. Under these conditions it is not surprising that the elderly are taken in by products claiming to slow down or reverse the aging process. Many companies exploit the fear of aging by making inaccurate, misleading, and unproven claims about their products. These claims are often based on questionable product testing. In 1986, consumers spent $1 to $2 billion on products claiming to prevent or remove wrinkles, restore skin softness, and alter other aspects of aging. This figure does not include the billions spent on cosmetic surgery.[28]

The production and sale of cosmetics is regulated by the Food and Drug Administration. By definition, cosmetics are substances intended to be rubbed, poured, sprinkled, or sprayed on the body to cleanse, beautify, promote attractiveness, or alter appearance. All ingredients making up more than 1 percent of a product must be listed on the label. Though manufacturers do have to document that products are safe, they do not have to prove that they work.

Cleansers and cold creams add moisture or promote moisture retention so the skin looks softer and smoother. Most contain water, and many also contain petroleum jelly and lanolin. Ingredients like vegetable oil and glycerine improve moisture retention. Alcohol may be added to enhance evaporation. There is no evidence that "special" ingredients like vitamin E, collagen, or estrogen will improve skin texture. There is also no evidence that more expensive products are any more effective than the "discount store" brands.

The purpose of skin bleaches is to fade dark spots due to freckles, moles, or liver spots. Skin treated in this way becomes sensitive to the sun, and the product label should note this. The FDA considers only one skin ingredient to be safe and effective. This is hydroquinone in concentrations of from 1.56 to 2.0 percent. *Consumer Reports,* after studying the effectiveness of fade creams, has made several observations:

1. If they work, it is only on freckles and age spots.

2. They do not cause blemishes to fade completely.

3. They should be applied only to dark areas.

4. Professional treatment should be considered if there are no results after three months.

5. The hands and face should be protected from the sun to prevent spots.

6. Make-up should be considered as an alternative for covering blemishes.[29]

Changes in the skin's appearance should be considered a natural part of growing older. Wrinkling results from loss of fluid and fat below the skin surface. The skin becomes less elastic and less supportive, causing the skin to "sag" slightly. In many older people it can actually enhance appearance by adding tremendous character and expression to the face. Although many cosmetics may claim otherwise, little can be done to prevent or remove wrinkles. To a great extent aging of the skin is determined by exposure to the sun in addition to factors like cigarette smoking and heredity.

Sun exposure is the major cause of premature wrinkles. Ultraviolet rays not only speed aging and wrinkling, but also increase the risk of certain types of cancer. Sun damaged skin is very wrinkled, thickened, and uneven in color. Consequently, the best protection for skin is to limit sun exposure as much as possible.

A number of products have been promoted for their supposed

abilities to slow aging or erase wrinkles. One of these products is vitamin E, sold in a number of forms: in cream form it sells quite well. However, research has indicated that vitamin E does not prevent or slow skin wrinkling. Some people, in fact, have had negative skin reactions to vitamin E cream.[30]

Hormone creams and collagen are other ingredients promoted for their anti-aging properties. These claims have never been proved, and have been disputed by respected and reputable sources. In fact, the Food and Drug Administration has stated that hormone creams are ineffective. Collagen, which contains a protein found in the white fibers of connective tissue, cartilage, and bone, may be added to cosmetics or injected directly under the skin by dermatologists. These injections are supposed to minimize or remove wrinkles. This procedure is costly and must be done several times. While collagen creams may soften skin, there is no evidence that they remove wrinkles. In addition, dermatology professor Dr. Marianne N. O'Donoghue has stated that procedures like tissue firming and collagen injections cannot enter the physiology of the skin or change skin permanently.[31]

Some alleged anti-aging products have been promoted by highly respected scientists. Glycel is a product claiming to contain a "rejuvenating ingredient" called glycosphingolipid (GSL). This product was endorsed by Dr. Christian Barnard, the surgeon who performed the first successful heart transplant. It sold for $75 a jar. However, dermatologist Dr. Vincent DeLeo has noted that it is only a moisturizer with a temporary effect on facial lines.[32]

Alfin Fragrances, Inc., which produced Glycel, was contacted by the Food and Drug Administration in 1988. A regulatory letter ordered the company to stop making anti-aging claims for its products. Similar letters were sent to Estee Lauder, Inc., Avon Products, Inc., and several other companies. The FDA noted that the anti-aging claims were illegal because the creams had not been proved safe and effective for their intended purposes.

It has even been claimed that some substances can extend life. Thirty-one chemicals were recommended by Dirk Pearson and Sandy Shaw in a book called *Life Extension*. Some are prescription drugs and some are vitamins and minerals naturally found in many foods. Several are potentially dangerous when taken in large doses. It is estimated that the treatment and tests recommended in *Life Extension* could cost up to $2000 a year.[33] The contents and thesis of Pearson and Shaw's book were reviewed by the U.S. House of Representatives Select Committee on Aging. The views of this committee were then summarized in a report. The report described the book as a "misinterpretation of sound aging research. . . . Isolated, unsubstantiated reports are used to validate hypotheses."[34]

There is no preparation or device on the market that can stop the aging process or extend the maximum life span in humans. However, over $2 billion is spent each year on anti-aging remedies.[35] To protect themselves, consumers need to question carefully what is seen and heard in advertisements. The National Institute on Aging has suggested several resources for elderly consumers concerned about their skin:

1. The American Academy of Dermatology
   930 N. Meacham Road
   Schaumburg, IL 60173-4965
   (708) 330-9830

   The academy represents dermatologists and provides pamphlets and referrals to the public.

2. The Skin Cancer Foundation
   245 Fifth Avenue, Suite 2402
   New York: NY 10016
   (212) 725-5176

   The foundaton works to promote awareness of the importance of early detection and treatment of skin cancer. It offers a variety of health education materials.

3. The National Institute on Aging Information Center
   P.O. Box 8057
   Gaithersburg, MD 20898-8057
   Request the reading: "Skin Care and Aging"

4. *Skin Secrets: A Dermatologist's Prescription for Beautiful Skin at Any Age,* by Joseph Bark. New York: McGraw-Hill, 1988.

GENERAL GUIDELINES

The National Institute on Aging has also suggested some general guidelines for defense against health quackery. The primary suggestions are to question all advertising and find out about a product or service before it is purchased. Some common ploys used by dishonest promoters are noted by the institute:

1. promising a quick or painless cure;

2. promoting a product made from a "special" or "secret" formula, usually available through the mail and only from one sponsor;

3. presenting testimonials or case histories from satisfied patients;

4. advertising a product as effective for a wide variety of ailments;

5. claiming to understand the cause or cure for a disease (such as arthritis or cancer) not yet understood by medical science.

ADDITIONAL RESOURCES

The following agencies can tell you of they have received complaints about a product or service. They can also offer advice about what to do if you have been a victim of quackery.

1. Council of Better Business Bureaus. This organization offers general advice on products and has worked with the Food and Drug Administration on two brochures: *Tips on Medical Quackery* and *Arthritis and Quackery and Unproven Remedies.* For free copies, send stamped, self-addressed envelopes for each brochure to:

   Council of Better Business Bureaus
   1515 Wilson Blvd.
   Arlington, VA22209
   Attn: Standards and Practices

2. The Food and Drug Administration (FDA). The FDA can answer questions about medical devices, medicines, and food supplements that are mislabeled, misrepresented, or harmful. Write:

   Food and Drug Administration
   HFE-BB, 5600 Fishers Lane
   Rockville, MD 20857

3. The U.S. Postal Service. The USPS monitors quack products purchased by mail. Write to:

   Postal Inspection Service
   Office of Criminal Investigation
   Washington, D.C. 20260-2166

4. The Federal Trade Commission (FTC). The FTC checks charges of false or deceptive advertising in publications or on the radio and television. Write:

Federal Trade Commission
6th St. and Pennsylvania Ave., NW.
Washington, DC 20580

NOTES

1. National Institute on Aging, "Aging Pages," United States Department of Health and Human Services (1985).

2. D. Benzaia, "The Misery Merchants," in *The Health Robbers,* 2d ed., edited by Stephen Barrett (Philadelphia: The George F. Stickley Co., 1980).

3. Food and Drug Administration. *A Study of Health Practices and Opinions.* #PB-210978 (Springfield, Va.: National Technical Information Services, U.S. Department of Commerce, 1972).

4. H. J. Cornacchia and S. Barrett, "Arthritis, Cancer, and AIDS," in *Consumer Health: A Guide to Intelligent Decisions* (St. Louis, Mo.: Times Mirror/ Mosby, 1989).

5. "FTC Challenges Health Claims of Mine Operator, Seeks Disclosure of Material Facts," *FTC News Summary,* no. 14, Washington, D.C. (June 28, 1974).

6. Benzaia, "The Misery Merchants."

7. Cornacchia and Barrett, "Arthritis, Cancer, and AIDS."

8. Arthritis Foundation, *Unproven Arthritis Remedies* (Atlanta, Ga.: The Foundation, 1987).

9. Cornacchia and Barrett, "Arthritis, Cancer, and AIDS."

10. Ibid.

11. Ibid.

12. M. L. Brigden, "Unorthodox Therapy and Your Cancer Patient," *Postgraduate Medicine* 81 (1987): 271–80.

13. Cornacchia and Barrett, "Arthritis, Cancer, and AIDS."

14. "Doctor Sentenced for Cancer Fraud," *Nutrition Forum* (May 1986), p. 1.

15. G. Radner, *It's Always Something* (New York: Simon & Schuster, 1989).

16. American Cancer Society, "Unproven Methods of Cancer Management: O. Carl Simonton, M.D.," *Ca—A Journal for Clinicians* 32 (1982): 59.

17. American Cancer Society, "Kelly Malignancy Index and Ecology Therapy," in *Unproven Methods of Cancer Management* (New York: The Society, 1971), pp. 127–29.

18. "Dentist Directed McQueen Therapy," *ADA News* (November 17, 1980): 1.

19. V. Herbert and S. Barrett, *Vitamins and "Health" Foods: The Great American Hustle* (Philadelphia: The George F. Stickley Co., 1981).

20. "Patients on Unproved Cancer Therapy Told How to Make Insurance Companies Pay," *Medical World News* (June 7, 1982).

21. Moertel, et al., "A Clinical Trial of Amygdalin Laetrile in the Treatment of Human Cancer," *New England Journal of Medicine* 42 (January 28, 1982): 201–206.

22. "Top Officials Cite Laetrile Dangers," *FDA Consumer* 11 (September 1977): 3–4.

23. V. Herbert, "Laetrile: The Cult of Cyanide," in *Nutrition Cultism: Facts and Fictions* (Philadelphia: The George F. Stickley Co., 1981).

24. Moertel, et al., "A Clinical Trial of Amygdalin Laetrile in the Treatment of Human Cancer."

25. "Laetrile: The Political Success of a Scientific Failure," *Consumer Reports,* 42 (August 1977): 444–47.

26. L. Lasagna, *Doctor's Dilemma* (New York: Harper and Row, 1962).

27. W. F. Janssen, "Cancer Quackery: Past and Present," *FDA Consumer,* 11 (July 1977): 27–32.

28. Cornacchia and Barrett, "Arthritis, Cancer, and AIDS."

29. "Fade Creams," *Consumer Reports,* 50 (January 1985): 12.

30. A. A. Fisher, "Cosmetic Warning: This Product May Be Detrimental to Your Purse," *Cutis,* 39 (January 1987): 23–24.

31. "Age-proofing Your Skin," *Health* 17 (September 1985): 40–42.

32. Fisher, "Cosmetic Warning: This Product May Be Detrimental to Your Purse."

33. Cornacchia and Barrett, "Arthritis, Cancer, and AIDS."

34. Report of the U.S. House of Representatives Select Committee on Aging.

35. "Age-proofing Your Skin."

ADDITIONAL REFERENCES

American Cancer Society, *Unproven Methods of Cancer Management* (New York: The Society, 1982).

G. A. Curt et al., "Immunoaugmentative Therapy: A Primer on the Perils of Unproven Treatment," *JAMA,* 255 (1986): 505–507.

10

Support for the Caregiver: Time Off without Guilt

Elizabeth A. Wegner

Giving care to an elder parent or being a helpful neighbor to an older adult can be a very difficult and frustrating job. Sometimes those who offer assistance experience feelings of helplessness, anger, inadequacy, fatigue, and in some cases they feel that a burden has been imposed on them. A burden has been defined as "the physical, psychological, emotional, social, and financial problems that can be experienced by family members caring for impaired older adults."[1]

Caregivers who are associated with an older adult have the heaviest responsibility of all. They are oftentimes the organizers of the elder's life and must decide if they want to perform a task themselves or hire someone to do it. It is the caregiver's responsibility to find out about available resources and about new developments and programs for older adults.

Women are the primary caregivers to older parents, and usually have little help in this task.[2] Women are more likely to become caregivers because they have performed caregiving tasks all their lives while taking care of children. While seeing to the needs of their elder adult(s) these women are being denied the opportunity to do something else, such as start a new job.[3] "Women in the Middle," those who have children and older parents to take care of, are constantly juggling their time. These women often experience role overload and jeopardize the fulfillment of their own basic needs.[4]

Psychologist Abraham Maslow defined four basic needs in life: *physiological, safety, love,* and *self-esteem.* Physiological needs are fulfilled through proper sleep and nutrition; safety needs are met if caregivers have security and order in their lives; love needs are fulfilled if supportive social relationships are encountered; and self-esteem refers to being happy with one's accomplishments and having self-respect.[5] These needs are especially important in caregiving, though not necessarily in the order given here.

Many needs of the caregiver can be lost through zealous caring for another person: for example, failure to maintain a proper diet or to get enough sleep. If the caregiver relies on the care receiver for money or housing, and the care receiver dies, basic physical needs may remain unfulfilled.

Safety needs may be a risk if the elder focuses on his or her impending death. This upsets the stability and security of both the caregiver and care receiver.[6] Depending upon the specific circumstances, the death of the elder could leave a void in the security of the caregiver and the surviving spouse of the deceased. The caregiver's lack of time to plan may diminish stability in his or her life. If the caregiver feels trapped by the situation and this leads to a feeling of not being in control, safety may be in jeopardy.

Love needs may be threatened if there is tension between the caregivers and elders who are related. Also, if the caregiver is forced to give up other commitments, for example, friendships or other relationships, love needs may not be fulfilled.[7]

The self-esteem of caregivers can be diminished if they feel that they may (or should) be able to help ease a disease process and are not doing so. Time constraints put on caregivers may cause activities in their own lives to be set aside or not given full attention, resulting in feelings of low self-esteem.[8] Also, if caregivers feel that they had no choice in becoming care providers, this may lead to resentment and a lack of confidence and competence.[9]

If one of the above basic needs is not fulfilled, a caregiving burden could result.

Many people take care of children throughout their lives, so caregiving is neither a new concept nor a new experience for them. But, when caring for an older adult, there are different crises. Five such situations are involved as the increased dependency of older adults distinguishes them from the dependency of children. These crises are: awareness of degeneration, unpredictability, time constraints, the caregiver-receiver relationship, and lack of choice.[10]

Children are raised in our society to become independent. Parents are full of pride when they see their children grow up and begin lives of their own. On the other hand, as older adults become more and more dependent, a caregiver may feel increased hopelessness and frustration.[11] This degeneration of an elder is a major crisis for potential caregivers.

The unpredictability in caring for an older adult contrasts sharply with the predictability of caring for a child. Child care decreases as the child ages, but care of an older adult may increase with age. Diseases found in older adults are often peculiar to each person. For example, a stroke or Alzheimer's disease in one person may have different effects in another person. To conclude, the future is tremendously unpredictable for those who care for older adults.[12]

Time constraints, the third crisis, is also a common problem for caregivers. When children are growing up, they are sent to school, which gives parents a little break. Daycare and baby-sitting are readily available to help share the care responsibilities. Caregiving to an older adult may not offer as many options. Services are available for people who need help caregiving, but they are not viewed as an accepted right.[13] Time constraints may be pushed to the limit of endurance if caregivers have their own family to take care of as well as a full- or part-time job.

The fourth crisis, the caregiver-receiver relationship, definitely changes as we age. Healthy families contain love and authority. Children are taught to obey their parents, and both parties show love to one another.[14] When caring for an older adult, the roles may be reversed. The new dependence of the parent on the child or younger adult may not be readily accepted. The love or friendship shown between them may be put to the test and conflicts may arise. Adult caregiving differs greatly from child rearing, in which the authority roles are established at beginning of life.[15]

The final crisis, lack of choice, is more of a problem with caring for older adults than caring for children. Many couples decide when to have children, and they have the choice of never having a family. On the other hand, there is little choice when the help of children is needed to care for aged parents. Caregivers may have to give up some of their personal and/or professional plans or take on tasks that they may not be able to or want to perform.[16] This situation is aggravated if caregivers have physical problems of their own.

The crises noted above may be damaging to the well-being of the caregiver. If the crises continue, help will be needed.

Views of the caregiving situation may differ depending upon the perspective of the caregiver or the care receiver. According to a study by Sandra J. Litvin, some general comments can be made.

Care receivers seem to have a more negative outlook on life than caregivers do. Also, care receivers see a conflict if they are unhappy or feel their relationship with the caregiver has somehow changed.[17]

Many older adults who receive care from a family member have lost a spouse and are grieving. Losing a spouse can be the most difficult hardship they may have to face. Also, the loss of friends can be very depressing. Many times, the adult children do not understand the loss felt by the older adult.[18]

Caregivers also perceive a conflict if the relationship with the care receiver has changed or if they feel the care receiver has reduced his or her activity with family or friends.[19] The caregiver's own responsibilities may dictate how they deal with the added stress of caring for an older adult.

Caregivers seemed to underestimate the care receiver's problems, both physical and social; the older adult's needs may not being met. This may be a way of shedding some of the guilt caregivers feel. If caregivers feel that older adults are healthy, both physically and socially, the burden of care may be lessened for a while.[20] It may be thought that any added help the elder may need can be avoided for the time being.

Many caregivers tend to underexpress the workload of caring for an elder parent. They do not want the parent to feel guilty for the help that is needed. Caregivers take on the added responsibility with little help from others in the family, and many times with little gratitude.

Both sides of the caregiving situation need to be examined further. Major life events and the lines of communication on each side can be factors in the amount of conflict that arises.[21]

Caregiving to an adult with a mental disorder can be even more difficult. "There is abundant evidence that caregivers to family members with a progressive dementia are more distressed than the general population."[22]

The death of a loved one who suffered from a mental disorder is upsetting but is often also a relief to caregivers. There are certain stages that the caregivers go through after losing a relative with a mental disorder.

First, the decline of the loved one somewhat prepares the caregiver psychologically for the death of the care receiver. Second, relief is felt when the caregiving responsibilities are lifted. Third, a year after the loved one has died, the feeling of guilt may resurface. "The greater the sense of loss during caregiving, the lower the depression during bereavement."[23]

According to Mullan, "Some interventions may be useful: Those that provide caregivers an opportunity to decrease their caregiver strains, to increase their sense of mastery, to feel less guilt about their caregiving, or to reflect on the losses they are experiencing."[24]

Interventions could include time away from the caregiving situation. Those who assist elders need time to accomplish tasks in their own lives and to relax. With all the responsibility that caregivers have, they may neglect themselves and their families. It is very important for them to have a break. Normal activities should not cease and time with their own families is necessary. For example, if the family takes a vacation every summer, they should continue this ritual. A home health aide or possibly a neighbor could be retained to stay with the elder for a few weeks. Many agencies are available that hire out part-time and full-time home health aides. Many of the aides have a Certified Nursing Assistant degree, and Licensed Practitioner Nurses can be hired if need be.

CASE STUDY

Mrs. Harmon, a forty-five-year-old school teacher, lives and works in Minnesota. Her parents reside only a few miles away in their own home. Recently, her parents have needed extra help doing daily activities around their house. Her father enjoys gardening, but needs help putting fertilizer on the garden. He is also a very good cook, but sometimes forgets certain recipes. Mrs. Harmon's mother enjoyed traveling, but cannot move about as easily, due to osteoporosis. She can still read to some extent, but her eyes are failing. Both of Mrs. Harmon's parents no longer drive, so she does most of it when the need arises. Mrs. Harmon has her own family to take care of, but fortunately her children are teenagers and do not require as much care.

One solution would be for all three of Mrs. Harmon's children to take turns driving their grandparents to certain destinations. Both parties very much enjoy spending time together. The grandchildren could also take turns cooking for their grandparents, and the grandparents could help the children with occasional spending money. The bond formed between the grandchildren and the grandparents would be strengthened as both elder and teen shape each others' lives in a special way.

CASE STUDY

Mr. and Mrs. Johnson live alone in a house in the country. They are not able to get to the grocery store very often and their respective arthritis conditions make cooking for themselves difficult.

A solution to this problem could be a great program called "Meals on Wheels." This meal service is in many cities and the food is delivered by volunteers. A hot meal is delivered to the older person's home at lunchtime. It contains one-third of the recommended daily allowance of nutrients and calories. The cost is kept low and affordable.

CASE STUDY

Dr. Parker, a physician and father in a small town, helps in the care of his older parents. He often finds himself torn between responsibilities to his family, his medical practice, and those involved with helping out with his parents. Dr. Parker has hired some home healthcare aides, but cannot overcome the guilt feelings he has when he is not able to be there for his parents. Dr. Parker decided to start a support group in his town.

Talking to others with the same problems can be a great help and a stress reliever. Support groups are formed specifically for that purpose. It is very important for frustrated caregivers to seek the help of a friendly ear. The burden of caregiving can become an overwhelming task, and without people who can listen and understand, caregivers may develop mental or physical problems. Depression or failure to take adequate care of themselves could be the unfortunate result.

Government help to caregivers is hard to assess. "Distress, in itself, is not a persuasive argument for resource allocation to groups by policymakers. Every group wanting support could express their discontent this way."[25] The fact that caregivers may disrupt their own lives or miss activities with their families is not a good enough argument for policy makers. The government seems to think that caregivers will exaggerate the problems to get support. In fact, caregivers feel loyalty and dedication to their care receivers, and tend to downplay their distress.[26] Becker and Morrissey observed this throughout an interview of caregivers who see to the needs of to Alzheimer patients.[27]

Despite patently depressed faces and vocal tone, our Alzheimer caregiver subjects would initially admit to only slight occasional . . . feelings of depression. But as the interview progressed with a systematic inquiry about depression-related symptoms, these same subjects would sometimes experience a very substantial welling of dysphoric affect denoting at least the presence of severe depressive emotion if not of depressive mood."[28]

Governments have enjoyed the public money saved if care can be accomplished in the home and by the family.[29]

Most of the time caregivers are family members who want to do everything possible to keep the elder out of a nursing home. The elder may become depressed at the thought of having to leave home. If the caregiving becomes too much of a burden, however, institutionalized care may become necessary. Caregivers have been able to find some comfort in respite programs, educational groups, and some new psychotherapeutic treatment provided by the government.

Rest and relaxation for caregivers is important for the physical and mental well-being of the entire family. A person in the caregiver role must know when to ask for help and to accept it when it is offered.

NOTES

1. L. George and L. Gwyther, "Caregiver Well-Being: A Multidimensional Examination of Family Caregivers of Demented Adults," *The Gerontologist* 26 (1986): 253–59.

2. E. M. Brody, . " 'Women in the Middle' and Family Help to Older People," *The Gerontologist* 21 (1981): 471–80.

3. V. Braithwaite, "Caregiving Burden; Making the Concept Scientifically Useful and Policy Relevant," 1992.

4. Ibid.

5. Ibid.

6. Ibid.

7. Ibid.

8. Ibid.

9. Ibid.

10. Ibid.

11. P. G. Archbold, "Impact of Parent-Caring on Women," *Family Relations* 32 (1983): 39–45.

12. R. F. Barnes, M. A. Raskind, M. Scott, and C. Murphy. "Problems of Families Caring for Alzheimer Patients: Use of a Support Group," *Journal of the American Geriatric Society* 29 (1981): 80–85.

13. Braithwaite, "Caregiving Burden; Making the Concept Scientifically Useful and Policy Relevant."

14. Ibid.

15. Ibid.

16. Ibid.

17. S. J. Litvin, "Status Transitions and Future Outlook as Determinants of Conflict: The Caregiver's and Care Receiver's Perspective," *The Gerontologist* 32 (1992): 68–76.

18. Ibid.

19. Ibid.

20. Ibid.

21. Ibid.

22. George and Gwyther, "Caregiver Well-Being: A Multidimensional Examination of Family Caregivers of Demented Adults."

23. J. T. Mullan, "The Bereaved Caregiver: A Prospective Study of Changes in Well-Being," *The Gerontologist* 32 (1992): 673–83.

24. Ibid.

25. Braithwaite, "Caregiving Burden; Making the Concept Scientifically Useful and Policy Relevant."

26. J. Becker and E. Morrissey, "Difficulties Assessing Depressive-like Reactions to Chronic Severe External Stress as Exemplified by Spouse Caregivers of Alzheimer Patients," *Psychology and Aging* 3 (1988): 300–306.

27. Ibid.

28. Braithwaite, "Caregiving Burden; Making the Concept Scientifically Useful and Policy Relevant."

29. Ibid.

11

Conclusion

Robert W. Buckingham, Dr. P.H.

I would like to end this volume with some words of advice for all who care for and care about the elders in our lives:

1. Be patient with your elder. Put yourself in his or her place. Ask yourself how you would like to be treated if the circumstances were reversed.

2. When you have concerns or questions, ask others how they have handled similar situations. Don't be afraid to collect a variety of opinions (even from health professionals) before you make a decision.

3. When things get tough or seem overwhelming, take a break—think—reflect. Sometimes it is necessary to remove yourself from the situation for a while. R + R + R is important (Rest + Reflect + Relax), then address the problem.

4. Have a sense of humor. Don't get so serious that you forget to laugh or smile. It will lighten your burden.

5. Incorporate your family or loved ones into the care process and the decision-making. Share the burden.

6. Expect to invest a great deal of time and energy in the relationship with your elder.

7. Don't allow the difficulty of the experience to load down your spirit. Use it to become more aware and sensitive.

8. Listen with an open mind and heart to what is going on around you.

9. Exercise the four dimensions of the human personality: physical, mental, emotional, and spiritual. Exercise them daily—

>   Physical—walking, running, bicycling, swimming, etc.
>   Mental—reading, analyzing, etc.
>   Emotional—learn to be patient, listen to others, open your heart
>   Spiritual—reflect, meditate, etc.

10. Balance your day: don't do too much of one thing.

11. Create a climate of growth for you and your elder.

12. Remember, a thousand-mile journey is taken one step at a time.

13. Do not try to become all things to all people. Take pride in your uniqueness.

14. Value what you and your elder are inside. Life is a matter of internals, not externals.

15. Enjoy the moment. Don't get wrapped up in the troubles of yesterday or the trials of tomorrow.

16. Be a light to others, not a judge.

17. Security, guidance, wisdom, and power are interlocking and interdependent. Security + guidance brings true wisdom. Wisdom becomes a spark to others to move forward toward personal growth and the power that it brings.

18. Let go of the anger, hurt, and pain from previous experiences and face today.

19. Remain confident in your beliefs.

20. The greatest tragedy in life is not sickness or death; the greatest tragedy is a life not fully lived. Make life your one great adventure!

Contributors

JAMES R. BEAL is a research assistant in the Department of Human Performance, Mankato State University, Mankato, Minnesota.

ROBERT W. BUCKINGHAM, Dr. P.H., is president of the Russian-American Institute of Health (Russian Academy of Sciences) and former dean of the College of Health and Human Performance at Mankato State University, Mankato, Minnesota.

KENNETH R. ECKER, Ph.D., is a professor in the Department of Human Performance, Mankato State University, Mankato, Minnesota.

PAUL M. GORDON, Ph.D., M.P.H., is a professor in the Department of Human Performance, Mankato State University, Mankato, Minnesota.

JAY KRUSE is a research assistant in the Department of Human Performance, Mankato State University, Mankato, Minnesota.

DAWN LARSEN, Ph.D., is a professor in the Department of Human Performance, Mankato State University, Mankato, Minnesota.

JENNIFER REMER is a research assistant in the Department of Human Performance, Mankato State University, Mankato, Minnesota.

ELIZABETH A. WEGNER is a research assistant in the Department of Human Performance, Mankato State University, Mankato, Minnesota.